PICKING UP THE PIECES

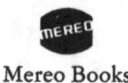

Mereo Books

2nd Floor, 6-8 Dyer Street, Cirencester, Gloucestershire, GL7 2PF
An imprint of Memoirs Books. www.mereobooks.com
and www.memoirsbooks.co.uk

PICKING UP THE PIECES
ISBN: 978-1-86151-851-4

First published in Great Britain in 2025
by Mereo Books, an imprint of Memoirs Books.

Copyright ©2025

Christine Redmond has asserted her right under the Copyright Designs and Patents Act 1988 to be identified as the author of this work.

A CIP catalogue record for this book is available from the British Library.
This book is sold subject to the condition that it shall not by way of trade or otherwise be lent, resold, hired out or otherwise circulated without the publisher's prior consent in any form of binding or cover, other than that in which it is published and without a similar condition, including this condition being imposed on the subsequent purchaser.

The address for Memoirs Books can be
found at www.mereobooks.com

Mereo Books Ltd. Reg. No. 12157152

Typeset in 11/17pt Garamond
by Wiltshire Associates.
Printed and bound in Great Britain

PICKING UP THE PIECES

Coping, caring and growth in
the midst of a pandemic

CHRISTINE REDMOND

Writing this book changed how I see life.

It gave me the courage to follow my heart and take steps toward the life I truly want. I hope you enjoy reading it. If any part of my story touches you, and you think I can help in some way, please feel free to reach out.

With love and thanks,
Christine

Email: chrissy@brave-coaching.co.uk
Facebook: Chris Redmond
Instagram: chrissy_redmond
www.brave-coaching.co.uk/download

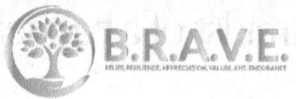

Contents

Chapter 1: *Picking up the pieces* 1
Chapter 2: *Origins* 6
Chapter 3: *A Calling Beyond* 15
Chapter 4: *Reflections Within* 26
Chapter 5: *In The Eye of the Storm* 34
Chapter 6: *Heartfelt Choices* 42
Chapter 7: *The Shadow of Sorrow* 51
Chapter 8: *Resilience and loss* 58
Chapter 9: *Finding Strength Through Reflection* 66
Chapter 10: *Embracing the Future* 73
Chapter 11: *Reclaiming Purpose* 88
Chapter 12: *Echoes of Change* 95
Chapter 13: *Bridges to Tomorrow* 103
Chapter 14: *The Power of Possibility* 110
Chapter 15: *Embracing the Journey* 124
            Epilogue: The Journey Continues 126

Preface

Life has a way of reshaping our paths when we least expect it. Sometimes it does it gently, nudging us towards a new direction. At other times it throws us into the deep end, forcing us to navigate waters we had never anticipated. For me, the latter was true. Just before the world was turned upside down by the 2020 COVID pandemic, I found myself facing a personal crisis—a relationship that crumbled unexpectedly, leaving me questioning everything I had once taken for granted. As I tried to regain my footing, the pandemic arrived, bringing with it unprecedented challenges, heartbreak, and ultimately, the devastating loss of a loved one.

At first, I did what many of us do—I pushed through, burying my emotions under the weight of responsibility. But as the months unfolded, I realised I couldn't simply carry on without addressing the storm raging inside me. I sought answers, delving into personal development, self-reflection, and the insights of those who had walked similar paths before me. What I discovered changed everything. Through this process, I uncovered a version of myself that was stronger, more resilient, and deeply attuned to the power of transformation.

This book began as a cathartic personal exercise—an attempt to put into words the emotions, lessons and revelations that surfaced during my journey. Initially, I started writing and reflecting on my experiences during the pandemic after being invited to contribute to a new book by Anthea Allen, a colleague who I had met after reading her first book, which was a compilation of emails sent to the community in London. What began as a single chapter soon evolved into something much greater—a deeply personal exploration that helped me make sense of all I had been through, an attempt to put into words the emotions, lessons, and revelations that surfaced during my journey. However, as the pages filled, I realised this wasn't just about me. My experiences, though deeply personal, mirror the struggles of so many others who have faced loss, uncertainty, and the daunting task of rebuilding a life that no longer looks the same.

My hope is that through sharing my story, others might find comfort, recognition, and perhaps even a roadmap to navigate their own challenges. This is a story of resilience, of breaking and rebuilding, of learning to embrace the unknown with courage. It is an invitation to those who find themselves at a crossroads—to step forward, not with fear, but with the quiet confidence that even in the darkest moments, transformation is possible.

Introduction

As I reflect on this journey, I am reminded of the immense challenges we all faced during Covid, the relentless battles both within and outside ourselves, and the profound transformations that emerged from those dark days. The pandemic tested the very limits of our endurance, forcing us to confront our deepest fears and vulnerabilities. It tore at the fabric of our lives, leaving scars that will forever remind us of the fragility and unpredictability of existence.

But within those scars lies a story of resilience, of a spirit that refused to be broken. My journey through the pandemic was not just about survival—it was about rediscovering the strength within, embracing the pain, and transforming it into a catalyst for growth. It was about learning that true healing comes not from running away from our emotions but from facing them head-on, with courage and compassion.

This book is more than a recounting of events; it is a testament to the power of resilience, the importance of self-compassion, and the transformative potential that lies within each of us. The experiences I've shared are deeply personal, yet I know they resonate with so many who have walked a similar path—those who have faced loss, uncertainty, and the overwhelming burden of responsibility.

As I look back on the journey, I am filled with a profound sense of gratitude for the lessons learned, for the growth that has come from adversity, and for the opportunity to now help others navigate their own challenges. The tools and practices that guided me through the darkest times—meditation, reflection, journaling—are now the foundations of my work as a mentor and teacher. They are the keys to unlocking the resilience within us all.

If you are about to read this book, my hope is that you will find within these pages not just a story of survival, but a guide to transformation. I hope you see the possibility of turning your own struggles into stepping stones for growth, and that you realise the immense power you hold to shape your life, no matter what challenges you face.

Remember, the journey of personal development is not a one-off event; it is a lifelong commitment to becoming the best version of yourself. It requires courage, persistence and a willingness to confront the uncomfortable truths within. But it is also a journey filled with immense rewards—clarity, purpose, and a deep sense of peace.

If you find yourself standing at a crossroads, unsure of the path ahead, know that you are not alone. There is a community of support, a network of individuals who have walked this path before you, ready to guide and uplift you. And I am here as your mentor, ready to walk alongside you, to share the tools and insights that have made all the difference in my life.

As we continue to heal from the scars left by the pandemic, let us carry forward the lessons learned, the resilience we have cultivated, and the unwavering belief that we can create a life filled with meaning, purpose, and love. Together, let us honour our journeys, embrace our growth, and step boldly into the future, ready to live a life we truly love.

CHAPTER 1

Picking up the pieces

I am sitting here considering what value I can add to a new book which is still being written. I met the author, Anthea Allen, for the first time last week. I contacted her after reading her wonderful first book, *Life, Death & Biscuits*, which is a compelling compilation of emails sent out to friends and neighbours during the pandemic. The book initially brought tears to my eyes, and I ended up sitting in a puddle as I re-lived the pandemic experience.

I am not a great believer in looking back – after all, why is the rear-view mirror so small and the windscreen so big?

It was a surprise to me that I had such an emotional reaction. Did I have PTSD? Why did I have that pain in my chest? Why was my heart beating so heavily? Why did I feel such deep sadness?

As the dust settled on the chaos of the pandemic, I

found myself grappling with the unseen scars left in its wake. Among these is the shadow of post-traumatic stress disorder (PTSD), a silent adversary lurking in the shadows of collective trauma endured. Flashbacks to harrowing moments, intrusive memories, that I thought had faded.

I sat with it and let my tears flow before I carried on. I could have chosen to hold it in, tell myself I was being ridiculous and ignore these overwhelming feelings, but time has taught me that if I acknowledge these emotions, sit with them and let them pass, then they will. It's when I bottle them up that they eventually explode in a dramatic outburst of anger, frustration and a complete meltdown. A bit like a hosepipe that has been blocked and eventually bursts.

I chatted with Anthea over a coffee as we shared experiences, scenarios we had faced and our challenges, but also our pride and gratitude for colleagues we had worked with. Anthea asked me if I would like to write a chapter for her next book. Of course I would! I was honoured.

The following day I pondered about what I might write, and started to read my journal for ideas. Wow! I had no idea that I had written in such detail about events that had taken place for me – us – and I remembered with mixed emotions of gratitude, sadness, appreciation and absolute disbelief what I – we – had all experienced.

It felt like a dream, as if it hadn't really happened, but it did, like a tsunami, with both barrels.

An inspired revelation emerged from my journaling practice that had come about from the personal development work I had started pre pandemic: the act of journaling became a pivotal tool in recognising my progress and triumphs. Through the lens of reflection, I connected the dots backwards, gaining insight into the strides I had made and the hurdles I had conquered. Without this practice, I might have viewed my experiences solely as a series of challenges to endure, rather than as significant milestones worthy of acknowledgment and celebration.

Suppressing my emotions at this time would have been like constructing barriers around myself, enclosing myself within a fortress of solitude. In order to fully embrace life's potential, I needed to confront and dismantle these self-imposed barriers that I thought I had overcome.

I have learnt that during times of intense pain and disbelief, it's tempting to sweep emotions under the rug, tucking them away in a corner of the mind. That is where they remain unless we find the tools to address and challenge these feelings; avoidance becomes our default coping mechanism. But turning a blind eye only delays the inevitable. In moments of profound pain and disbelief, I often found myself burying my emotions, tucking them away in the shadowy corners of my mind. I convinced myself that out of sight meant out of heart and mind, but deep down, I knew those unacknowledged feelings were still there, waiting for me to face them. Without the tools to process and challenge what I was feeling, avoidance became my default response—a reflective shield that ultimately deepened my inner struggles. Ignoring the whispers of my turmoil only delayed the inevitable reckoning, turning a fleeting escape into a heavier, more burdensome weight. I learned that true healing begins only when I summon the courage to uncover what I had hidden and confront the truths I had long ignored.

It's like a trip switch waiting to be triggered. I knew this, yet still these emotions raised their heads once again. A stark reminder that working on oneself is something to be carried out consistently if true healing is to take place.

I thought I had continued to work on myself, hence the surprise of my reaction. This is what has driven me to write this short book. It's a cathartic experience for me and if it resonates with anyone and helps them to accept, move on or just dive deeper into their life and emotions, then I am happy to share as far and wide as possible. No matter what we might feel sometimes, alone, isolated or misunderstood, I am willing to bet that someone else has been through, or is going through, exactly the same thing. You are never alone, and I wish to hold out a branch to anyone who feels they are.

The past has a way of revealing itself when we least expect it. What I believed to be neatly tucked away resurfaced with full force, reminding me that healing is not a destination but an ongoing journey. A simple conversation, a moment of reflection, or even reading another's words can unlock emotions we thought were long buried. Acknowledging these feelings—rather than suppressing them—became a turning point for me, reinforcing the power of self-awareness and emotional mastery. Through journaling, introspection, and allowing myself to sit with discomfort, I began to see the lessons within the pain. But every journey has a starting point, a moment where life shifts, sometimes opening us up to something new. In the next chapter, I revisit the moment my personal world cracked—the relationship breakdown that became the catalyst for my transformation, setting me on a path I had never seen coming.

CHAPTER 2

Origins

My journey started back in 2019 when I suffered a relationship breakdown; I say 'suffered' because it hurt, a lot. I didn't see it coming and it put me into quite a dark place in my personal life. I was the Matron of an Intensive Care Unit (ITU) and loved my job. Surrounded by colleagues, patients and families, I diligently carried on with my day job whilst feeling broken inside. I never really shared this experience with others, except for a few close colleagues, as I felt embarrassed, angry, ashamed and a failure, so as far as everyone was aware it was business as usual.

As I delve into the complexities of my feelings surrounding the relationship breakdown and the profound connection I feel to nursing, I need to provide insight into my upbringing and the ingrained notions of societal expectations that shaped my perspective into adulthood.

I was raised in the Catholic faith, immersed in principles that were not just taught but woven into the fabric of my upbringing. These beliefs were passed down through my family and childhood, forming the foundation of the way I saw the world and my place within it. They shaped my sense of identity and, in many ways, dictated how I navigated life's challenges—especially when it came to relationships.

Growing up, I absorbed the unspoken rule that relationships and marriage are sacred, lifelong commitments. This idea wasn't questioned; it was simply the truth as I understood it. When my first marriage ended, I was already carrying the weight of what I perceived as failure, but the collapse of a second significant relationship compounded those feelings. Even without the formalities of marriage in this case, the commitment was just as real to me, just as binding.

These deeply rooted beliefs about family and relationships became a lens through which I judged myself – harshly. I didn't stop to question whether these ideals still resonated with the person I had become as an adult. Instead, I internalised them as evidence of my own inadequacy, leaving me to wrestle with feelings of failure and self-doubt. It wasn't just the end of the relationship I was mourning—it was the loss of the person I believed I was supposed to be.

During my childhood, I was naturally inclined towards sensitivity and caring qualities which would shape both my character and my destiny in profound ways.

I come from a family of four girls, of whom I am the third. Our parents were hard-working people, and our formative years, until I reached the age of ten, were spent in a modest council estate in West London. It was during this time that my parents realised their dream of acquiring a home of their own, and I can still recall the sheer excitement that coursed through me. This was rooted in several things. First and foremost, we had a house, complete with a garden which I envisaged would serve as a safe haven for our playtime. The environment we had been raised in so far was not unsafe by any means, but I had always felt like a bit of an outsider.

Our new home was a cosy three-bedroom semi-detached house, with a modest garden that backed onto open fields. It held a simple charm, offering a sense of warmth and possibility. I can vividly recall helping my dad decorating, holding up strips of wallpaper as he carefully measured and cut them, ensuring each pattern lined up just so. The scent of wallpaper paste filled the air, mingling with the quiet focus of those shared moments.

In the garden, we claimed a small patch of soil for growing vegetables, surrounding it with a quaint white picket fence to keep it safe from wandering feet. Together, we prepared the earth, planting seeds with care and anticipation. The first signs of life breaking through the soil felt like tiny victories, and the taste of our homegrown vegetables remains a vivid memory—fresh, crisp, and steeped in the love that had nurtured them.

Those early days shaped more than just my surroundings; they laid the foundation for the way I would later create a home of my own. Even now, as I plan my vegetable patch each year, the rhythm of planting, growing, and harvesting brings me back to that garden, to the feeling of connection and care that made our house truly a home.

Our family also welcomed a new member, Lady, our black crossbred dog, affectionately referred to as a "Heinz 57" after a brand that was then a household name. There was no need for fancy crossbreed titles back then. Additionally, I took on the responsibility of caring for a cat, Penny, whenever her elderly lady owner next door was away. Penny was a soft, loving tortoiseshell cat who adored cuddles and affection. While the rest of my family remained relatively indifferent to her, I cherished our time together. Each time I cared for Penny, she would inevitably present me with a mouse, a gesture which always brought a smile to my face, thanks to my mother's insistence that it was a gift.

My parents, both Irish, had come to England in their late teens to build a life and start a family. Our home was often filled with the warmth of visiting family, especially when our grandmothers came to stay. I always looked forward to their visits—it felt like a little celebration every time they were with us. One of my favourite rituals was bringing them tea in the mornings, carefully balancing the tray as I knocked on their door. I'd sit with them, savouring those quiet moments of conversation, listening to their stories and soaking up their gentle wisdom. It was during those cherished visits that I first discovered the joy of caring for others. I still recall one of my nanas smiling at me and saying, almost as if she could see my future laid out before me, that I'd make a wonderful nurse someday. Those words stayed with me, quietly taking root in my heart, shaping the path I would eventually follow.

As a sensitive child, my sisters often engaged me in various "games" that frequently concluded with me in tears while they erupted into laughter, something they still remember and refer to even today. But that's a story for another time. Although I may not always outwardly display it now, I have come to embrace and acknowledge my enduring sensitivity as an integral part of who I am. I have also learned how to harness it to my advantage, channelling that sensitivity into my dedication to understanding and serving others.

While my sisters effortlessly bonded with the neighbouring children upstairs, I found myself left with a solitary connection to the young boy of the family. Despite the warmth of our home, this arrangement left me yearning for a deeper sense of belonging and companionship.

I can't say I ever really enjoyed school and I have limited memories of it. However, I distinctly remember an annual careers day. I seized the opportunity to speak with a gentleman who had enquired about my aspirations for adulthood. Without hesitation, I expressed my desire to become a nurse. While these memories of my early school years are somewhat hazy, I vividly recall his response: "All little girls say they want to be a nurse. It's poorly paid and involves unsocial hours. Now, what do you really want to do?" I can't recall the specifics of how that conversation unfolded, but I do know that his words cast immediate doubt in my mind, convincing me that nursing wasn't a worthwhile pursuit. Or so I believed at the time.

Upon completing my schooling, I found myself employed in the cargo section of an airline. My responsibilities were primarily administrative, involving cargo bookings, manifest completion, and the intricacies of handling hazardous cargo, including packaging and documentation compliance to ensure safety regulations were met.

Ironically, this job demanded shift work, including night shifts, mirroring one of the very reasons I had initially dismissed a career in nursing. I remained in this role for a few years before transitioning to a freight forwarding company, where I eventually met my husband.

My journey continued as I married and welcomed three beautiful children into my life, all while juggling part-time administrative roles that failed to ignite any real passion within me. Nevertheless, they provided a means to support my family while allowing me to care for my children.

Just before my daughter embarked on her educational journey, I found myself contemplating my own future. I had a lingering itch that demanded my attention—something deep within urging me to pursue more—and it needed to be scratched. I felt a pull toward nursing, a field I'd long admired, and began to consider the possibility of turning that pull into a purpose. Although I already held the necessary qualifications, I hadn't studied in many years and wasn't entirely sure whether I had the capacity—mentally or practically—to commit to a full three-year degree. So, as a test to myself, I enrolled in an access to nursing course. It was the stepping stone I needed, a way to dip my toes in without fully diving. To my surprise, I found myself thoroughly enjoying it—the mental stimulation, the structured learning, and the camaraderie of other mature students who, like me, were returning to education after life had taken them in different directions. That experience reaffirmed my decision, and soon after, I was accepted into a university nursing programme—just as my daughter took her first steps into school. Two parallel journeys were beginning, hers and mine.

Back in those days, nurses were fortunate enough to receive a bursary to support their education. Our training was aligned with school holidays, a detail that, with the support of my family and my husband, allowed me to pursue my dream. Reflecting upon those years, I can say that they were demanding. Balancing nurse training with the responsibilities of raising three vibrant children presented numerous challenges, but I wouldn't trade that experience for anything in the world.

> *The end of a relationship is never just about two people going their separate ways—it's an unravelling of identity, a confrontation with deeply ingrained beliefs, and often, a painful mirror reflecting the doubts and insecurities we've carried all along. In my case, the heartbreak I experienced wasn't just about loss—it was about the collision of my past conditioning with my present reality. The expectations I had grown up with clashed with the truth of who I was becoming, leaving me questioning everything. But, painful as it was, this breaking point became a catalyst for something greater. It forced me to look inward, to challenge the narratives I had accepted as truth, and to ask myself who I truly was beyond the roles I had played. This was the beginning of a transformation that would lead me to a deeper understanding*

of my purpose—not just in my personal life, but in my career. In the next chapter, I explore how my calling to serve others extended far beyond what I had imagined, and how I came to realise that healing—both my own and that of those around me—was at the heart of my journey.

CHAPTER 3

A Calling Beyond

My upbringing, characterised by sensitivity, empathy and a natural inclination to care for others, coupled with the trials and tribulations I faced along the way, ultimately propelled me toward the nursing profession. It was a journey guided by love, driven by a deep sense of purpose, and unwavering determination. Today, I stand as a testament to the power of resilience and the boundless potential within us all, despite the odds and recommendations that once stood in my path.

I have learnt that pursuing your dreams, even in the face of misunderstanding, holds a profound significance. Too often, we allow logical reasoning, fear and limiting beliefs (all food for the mind) to dictate our paths, yet rarely does the mind hold a more accurate or truthful compass than the heart. In navigating life's choices, coherence between the head and heart is paramount. Because they are the two sides of the same decision-making coin, if they're in conflict, then so are you.

As a nurse, the essence of giving and caring goes beyond mere professionalism; it becomes a vocation, an intrinsic part of one's being. Nursing isn't just a job title; it's a way of life, a calling that defines who you are. This commitment to compassion and service extends beyond the confines of a clock, for it is woven into the fabric of your very existence. It's the distinction between fulfilling a duty and answering a higher calling.

Have you ever had that experience when something you are doing feels so natural, so right?

Where despite the challenges you may be facing, you know with all your heart this is exactly where you are meant to be?

Throughout my career, I've always been driven by a profound desire to help others, initially believing that nursing was my destined path in life. However, in recent years, I've discovered that this inclination, coupled with the valuable skills I've nurtured, has not only elevated me to the pinnacle of my nursing profession but opened doors to a fulfilling career as a trainer, a personal coach and mentor. This journey has taught me that while I may be ready to move away from the clinical aspects of nursing, the fundamental essence of the profession—compassion and service—remains deeply woven into every aspect of my work. Whether I'm providing hands-on care in a hospital setting or guiding clients as a coach, these core principles continue to shape my identity and role within the healthcare world. This realisation has resulted in a pivotal shift in my perspective, illustrating that the heart of nursing can extend far beyond traditional clinical roles and enrich other pathways, including personal coaching.

Now that you have a glimpse into my background and understand why nursing holds a special place in my heart, let's shift back and return to the topic at hand: the relationship breakdown.

I struggle to leave situations gracefully, because I often find it challenging to enter them with ease. The difficulty in letting go stems from a deeper struggle with forming attachments and embracing love. Reflecting on the intense moments of my adult life, I've come to realise that they trace back to beliefs I internalised in childhood.

Self-doubt and feelings of not being good enough had a huge part to play in this. These deeply ingrained patterns have influenced my approach to relationships, complicating the process of dissolution and navigating through the aftermath of a breakdown. Through introspection and self-awareness, I've begun to dismantle these pre-installed patterns, forging a path toward growth and healing.

I found myself consumed by questions that refused to let go. What was it about human psychology that allowed some people to rise above their challenges, achieving so much, while others, like me, seemed trapped in an endless cycle of grief, pain, and sadness? What did they know that I didn't? What inner strength or wisdom did they possess that seemed so elusive to me? And most pressing of all—how was I going to break free from this heaviness? How was I going to find my way back to a life that felt worth living? The need to uncover these answers ignited a burning curiosity within me, a longing to understand and, ultimately, to heal.

The introspection and self-awareness I developed were the first steps in taking a proactive approach to navigating this challenging time. I enrolled in numerous personal development courses, eventually finding one that, though I didn't realise it at the time, may very well have saved my life. Even more transformative were the few close, special friends and family members who stood by me. It's undeniable—the people you choose to surround yourself with have the greatest impact on your life. In moments like these, true friends don't just step up; they show up in ways that leave an indelible mark on your heart and your journey forward.

As is usually the case with such things, the course that changed my life was not the first one I found. I spent a lot of time, money and energy scouring the web for what I needed. The one I initially stepped into was the Robbins Madanes Core 100 coaching course, in October 2019. While this course is incredible, it wasn't the one that changed my life because, as I was about to discover, it was the right thing at the wrong time.

I was drawn to coaching, as I always knew I liked to support people. After 24 years I'd reached a point where I thought I had achieved my life goal by doing that through nursing. To a certain degree I did, but this was an achievement that was now behind me. I reached my ultimate goal of becoming a nursing specialist, which felt good, but I knew I had more to give somewhere. It's like dreaming about something and saying to yourself, *"if only I could.... then I would be happy or content or fulfilled"*. You are, I was, these things for a short moment in time, but then I wanted something else, and so the wheel goes round.

I remember thinking that if I could just get through university and secure my degree and then a job I loved, I would be sorted. If that had happened though I would have been bored, stagnant. We all need something to be striving for.

Looking back, I realise that, much like plants, our existence hinges on growth and contribution to thrive. Every living being, including ourselves, follows this fundamental principle; if we're not actively growing, we're stagnating, slowly withering away. Just as neglecting to water a flower impedes its ability to contribute to the environment and eventually leads to its demise, failing to nurture our own growth stifles our potential and diminishes our impact on the world around us.

After just a few months, I paused my initial Robbins Madanes Core 100 coaching training. I had realised I was one of the people who needed the very interventions we were being taught. How could I ever offer this to someone else if I couldn't do it for myself?

I knew I had to do some work on myself prior to helping others. I realised that I needed to heal the wounds I carried from the relationship breakdown, and that if I didn't I would forever be limited in what I could offer others and how much joy I could find in my own life.

However, there was one Tony Robbins quote which really landed with me: "What would happen if you just put it down? Shoot it to the moon!"

Hearing this touched something inside. I asked myself, "What am I not putting down?"

I reflected upon this, looking inside to identify what I was holding onto that was keeping me stuck to this situation.

Tony Robbins then asked, "What happens if you do, what happens if you don't?"

I couldn't escape my thoughts, holding onto the pain I was telling myself I was so desperate to move beyond. Could it be as easy as choosing something different?

This confirmed what I knew: that I needed to take a step back and bring greater focus to working on myself.

Reflecting on my journey, I now see how this particular course became a pivotal catalyst, leading me to my ultimate transformational mentor. This mentor opened my eyes to the intricacies of quantum physics, revealing a profound truth: life responds to the intentions we set with our minds.

It was a revelation to learn that not all thoughts are inherently true; they are constructs of the mind, shaped by perception. More importantly, I came to understand that thoughts act as pathways for energy, and the direction of that energy shapes our reality. This insight underscored the power of choosing where to focus. As one of my mentors often says, "Where focus goes, energy flows." This became evident when I enrolled in the Robbins Madanes Core 100 coaching training. I was eager to help others, but I soon realised that I first needed to work on myself. My energy had been directed outward, seeking to support others while neglecting my own healing. Recognising this, I shifted my focus inward, prioritising my personal growth. This decision not only transformed my own life but made me a more effective mentor. It reinforced a powerful truth: when we focus on healing and self-development, transformation naturally follows.

In the realm of personal development, there's a certain truth in the saying, "When you know, you know."

It reflects those moments of clarity when we recognise our readiness for transformation. Similarly, the adage "When the student is ready, the teacher appears" holds a deep meaning. At key points in our lives, when we are truly open to growth, the right mentor or guide often emerges—offering the wisdom and support needed to navigate uncharted paths. This moment of readiness, combined with the guidance of a mentor, became the foundation of my own transformation.

Sometimes, we need someone to stand by our side, providing insight and encouragement as we step across the threshold into a new phase of life. This guide or teacher helps illuminate our path, offering perspectives and tools that align with our evolving needs. Their presence is not just about imparting knowledge but about walking with us as we integrate new understanding and embark on transformative journeys. For me, this came when I discovered Peter Sage's Elite Mentorship Forum. At a time when I felt lost, his teachings provided a framework that challenged my long-held beliefs and reshaped my perspective. Through his mentorship, I learned to harness the power of my thoughts, shift my mindset and reclaim control over my life. Similarly, in the early days of the pandemic, the consultant I worked with in intensive care became a source of unwavering support. His expertise and calm leadership provided a much-needed anchor during the chaos, helping me navigate the immense pressures we faced.

In these moments, the guidance we receive can be pivotal, enabling us to embrace change with confidence and move forward with a deeper sense of purpose and direction.

My journey towards true transformation commenced in January 2020 when I met my aforementioned mentor, Peter Sage, and embarked on a transformative experience as he guided me through his award-winning Elite Mentorship Forum, considered by many to be the gold standard in personal development.

My first experience with his training came when I participated in a five-day challenge led by Peter. I embarked on a deep dive into my true vision, challenged my self-limiting beliefs, and scrutinised my thought patterns.

Through dedicated practice, I honed the ability to confront and overcome negative thoughts, fundamentally altering my perspective on life. My study with Peter allowed me to truly cherish the wisdom encapsulated in one of my favourite quotes by Dr. Wayne Dyer: "If you change the way you look at things, the things you look at change." This mantra serves as a constant reminder of the transformative power of perspective, and how when we change the context, we can change our life. We can completely change our experiences of life by adopting a context of positivity and possibility.

It's a phrase I carry with me, grounding me in moments of doubt and uncertainty, instilling within me the resilience to navigate life's twists and turns with grace and optimism. To this day, in fact only today, I have had to remind myself of this and change my perspective on something that happened.

I had a situation at work that would potentially mean having to do a different job. I found myself going down a spiral of negative thoughts and emotions, what ifs, and filling in the blanks with worst case scenarios. I had to stop myself in my tracks: this could be a blessing, it could give me time to really work on things that are close to my heart. I concluded with the thought, 'if it's not this it will be something better'. I know many people who have lost their job, had to transfer somewhere else or been forced to leave because their work environment has become intolerable, yet would say today that it was the best thing that could have happened to them, because it allowed them to embrace a new and more positive direction in life.

This work is not a one-time effort; it's a lifelong commitment, a way of being that demands consistency and care to truly take root. Once again, I was reminded that growth isn't achieved through a single breakthrough but through the daily, intentional practice of nurturing these principles. It's in showing up, day after day, that this work becomes not just something you do, but a part of who you are. True embodiment requires devotion, persistence, and the understanding that transformation is a journey, not a destination.

> *Nursing was never just a profession for me—it was a calling, an innate drive to serve, to care, and to make a difference in people's lives. But as I navigated my own personal struggles, I began to see that this calling extended beyond the walls of the hospital. The same qualities that made me a compassionate nurse—empathy, resilience, and an ability to guide others through difficult moments—were leading me toward something even greater. My journey into personal development didn't just help me heal; it opened my eyes to a deeper truth about the human experience. I realised that the way we see the world isn't just shaped by external circumstances—it is a direct reflection of our inner state. This realisation was transformative. If my outer world was a mirror of my inner world, then true change had to start from within. This understanding, though powerful, was only the beginning.*
>
> *In the next chapter, I explore how this shift in perspective reshaped my reality and became the foundation for lasting transformation.*

CHAPTER 4

Reflections Within

There were many profound and life-changing moments as I continued my journey through the Elite Mentorship Forum. One of the most profound realisations I gleaned from this experience was the concept that your outer world follows your inner world.

What does this entail? It means that how you perceive and interpret the external reality is deeply intertwined with your internal state of being. In essence, your inner state provides the lens through which you view your outer world.

What does that even mean? The external circumstances and experiences in your life are influenced by your thoughts, beliefs, emotions and attitudes. In other words, what you think, feel, and believe internally shapes and manifests in your external reality.

And what does that mean? Well, for me personally if I

hold onto positive thoughts, maintain a hopeful attitude, and believe in my abilities, I'm more likely to attract positive experiences and opportunities in my life. Conversely, if I constantly dwell on negative thoughts, hold onto fear or doubt, and have a pessimistic outlook, I may find myself encountering more challenges or negative outcomes.

A powerful moment of clarity came when I realised that my sense of burnout and frustration in my professional life was not just due to external pressures but also my internal struggle with self-worth and boundaries. The more I nurtured resilience and self-compassion, the more I found strength in my work and purpose in my challenges. This shift reinforced a simple but life-altering lesson: transformation begins within. If I wanted to create change in my outer world, I had to first cultivate it internally.

This concept is often associated with the idea of the law of attraction, which suggests that like attracts like, and that your thoughts and emotions have the power to attract corresponding experiences into your life. Therefore, by cultivating a positive inner world characterised by optimism, gratitude, and self-belief, you can create a more positive and fulfilling outer world. It's an example of a self-fulfilling prophecy.

This insight was immensely empowering, as it highlighted the fact that any efforts to enhance my life must first begin with cultivating my inner sense of fulfilment and well-being. Looking back, I began to notice how this dynamic played out in others too—although, prior to developing a deeper understanding of how the outer world mirrors the inner world, I likely wouldn't have recognised it for what it was. I recall one nurse on the unit who was clearly struggling. She had become withdrawn, disengaged, and was taking frequent periods of sick leave. When I sat down with her, she opened up about feeling deeply homesick and uncertain about her future, and admitted she was considering leaving altogether. Rather than lose a good nurse to burnout and overwhelm, we explored her options together. With the support of my manager, we arranged a three-month sabbatical, incorporating a small amount of unpaid leave and ensuring she still had at least a week of annual leave remaining upon her return. This was intentional—not for immediate use, but to give her the flexibility to take another break later in the year, helping to protect her well-being and avoid sliding back into the same place. The transformation when she returned was remarkable. She was lighter, more focused, and visibly happier. She had clarity about her next steps and soon after began a short-term role with the practice educator, where she flourished. It was a clear and powerful example of how giving someone the space to realign internally can lead to a complete shift in how they show up in the world around them.

There is the story of a man who lost his car keys inside his house. Despite thoroughly searching every room, he couldn't find them. Frustrated and despairing, he decided to step outside into the garden and take a break with a cup of tea. It was only then, as he relaxed in the sunshine, that he remembered he had left them in his car when he had been unloading it earlier. The point of the story is that sometimes, when faced with challenges or obstacles, we need to shift our perspective to find solutions. By stepping into the light, both literally and metaphorically, we can gain new insights that enable us to overcome difficulties more effectively.

This story emphasises the importance of openness to different viewpoints and the power of changing our environment to change our perception of a situation.

I found that developing positive habits requires both determination and consistent practice, along with the support of like-minded individuals to keep me accountable and motivated along the way. The journey towards cultivating these habits is not without its challenges; indeed, it is often fraught with tests and trials.

However, it is through recognising and embracing these challenges, and staying steadfast in my commitment, that I began to witness meaningful change unfold in my life.

Consistency in your actions, coupled with a resilient mindset, paves the way for transformative growth and lasting success.

This marked a seminal moment in my life, as powerful insights were gained and new empowering perspectives were adopted. Things I had never considered to be possible now seemed to be available to me. But I would still ask myself – am I really the master of my own life? It didn't feel like it. I felt as though I was merely reacting to everything that happened to me, as though I had absolutely no control, being pulled from here to there in a crazy and unpredictable way like a paper bag in a gale.

Have you ever unconsciously reacted to something, only to regret your actions when looking back in hindsight? I know I did, quite often, and sometimes so much so that I felt compelled to go back and apologise.

I used to judge myself for this, confused as to how I could so easily slip into this behaviour, all the time blind to the fact that this is a very common part of the human experience, and something that we resolve by doing our inner work.

The timing of my finding Peter Sage was perfectly synergetic, arriving in the ideal moment. And what is incredible is that I had only just consumed the first few modules before they began to play a pivotal role in my life.

In retrospect, I realise that my encounter with Peter wasn't merely coincidental and due to the circumstances of my relationship. Rather, it was essential preparation, a precursor to the profound upheaval that was on the brink of engulfing the world. It's proved to be a great example of everything happening for a reason.

I began to cultivate an awareness of my thoughts, capturing them in my journal whenever I could. Each entry became a reflection of my day and a quiet declaration of what I hoped for on the next. A key part of this practice was listing the things I felt grateful for—a ritual that brought moments of comfort and lightness. At the time, I saw it as a pleasant exercise, as I didn't yet grasp the true depth of its power. It was only later that I realised how this simple act of gratitude was quietly shaping my perspective, helping me shift from merely surviving to embracing life with renewed purpose and hope.

I don't think I would have got through the year without these things and it's only with the benefit of hindsight that I now see their true worth. These journals kept me in a relatively positive space. I would write about my experiences but would always end with a positive goal and intention for the following day based on my reflections of the day gone by.

However, when faced with intense challenges, I found myself abandoning many of the personal development tools I had worked so hard to acquire. Meditation, which I had only just begun to practise, became less frequent, leaving space for self-doubt to creep in. At first, I questioned whether this path was truly meant for me. Was personal development just a fleeting distraction, something that offered temporary comfort but no real transformation? These doubts lingered, making me wonder if I had misunderstood the journey altogether—or if I simply wasn't ready to fully commit to it.

It seems it's a common human tendency to appreciate the value of something only when it's gone—a lesson echoed by many personal development teachers, who often emphasise the importance of seizing opportunities for growth and self-improvement before they slip away unnoticed.

In hindsight, my interaction with Peter and the self-improvement skills I acquired were essential groundwork for the gathering storm that was about to unfold, the importance of which, once again, I only later understood.

> *As I peeled back the layers of my inner world, I discovered that true transformation begins within. The connection between my thoughts and reality became undeniable, guiding me towards a deeper sense of self-awareness. But awareness alone was not enough. I had to learn how to implement this understanding, to reshape my responses, to let go of deeply ingrained fears that had long dictated my life. This realisation was empowering but also overwhelming—what would it truly mean to take ownership of my life? And could I hold onto these in-*

sights when tested by external forces beyond my control?

In the next chapter, this newfound clarity is put to the ultimate test as the world outside descends into unprecedented chaos, challenging everything I thought I had learned.

CHAPTER 5

In The Eye of the Storm

Now let us step into March 2020, when the world stood on the precipice of an unprecedented crisis as the COVID-19 pandemic rapidly spread across the globe.

Governments and healthcare systems scrambled to contain the outbreak, yet uncertainty loomed large. In the United Kingdom, bustling streets and vibrant city centres at first retained an air of normality, albeit tinged with an underlying sense of apprehension. Businesses operated, schools were open, and social gatherings persisted, but whispers of caution grew louder with each passing day. International travel waned, and news headlines were dominated by rising infection rates and mounting casualties.

People cautiously navigated their daily routines, listening to the daily news reports on the number of deaths. We saw people stocking up on essentials and adopting newfound hygiene practices. Little did everyone know that in a matter of days, the nation would be plunged into a historic lockdown, reshaping life as they knew it and underscoring the fragility of human existence in the face of an invisible adversary.

In my hospital we had some knowledge about the SARS-CoV-2 virus, but like everyone else we found ourselves firefighting in the hospital. We started to see an influx of patients and I recall walking around our 15-bedded intensive care unit with the consultant designing antechambers, transitional spaces for people to put on and take off protective clothing prior to going into the main area that would be used to nurse these highly infectious patients.

We had a team of people put up structures built from wooden frames and plastic sheeting that allowed us to don and doff our protective clothing. 'Don' and 'doff', words with ancient roots which are rarely used in modern conversation, were not terms you would hear much in healthcare circles either before the pandemic, but they had now become part of our everyday language.

I remember thinking this was madness. Was it really going to be necessary to have these chambers? If it was, then surely we needed something somewhat more advanced than our Blue Peter designs. It felt like something out of MASH, the 1970s TV series centred around interrelationships, stress and trauma involved in being a part of a Mobile Surgical Army Hospital.

We were neither architects nor designers—simply a doctor and a nurse doing our utmost to find solutions that would ensure everyone's safety. My consultant was absolutely remarkable; his knowledge of airflow and ventilation was extraordinary. He had meticulously studied every detail and brought an incredible depth of expertise to the situation.

Staff came in on their days off to help convert ordinary wards into temporary intensive care units. This involved contractors who came to install additional electrical sockets for the amount of equipment we needed to use.

We chuckled nervously as the electricians informed us that installing the necessary sockets would take a week, as we were fully aware that this task needed completion within 24 hours. Undeterred, we conveyed the urgency of the situation to them. To our amazement, they embarked on the challenge with unwavering determination. Their tireless efforts and commitment were nothing short of heroic as they worked relentlessly to meet the deadline. In a heartening display of solidarity, nurses rallied around them, offering tea and cakes to fuel their endeavours as they laboured to accomplish their mission.

Our practice educator, who also happened to be my partner in crime on the unit, organised training sessions for the entire staff. We had multiple sessions daily, dedicated to the fine art of donning and doffing our protective gear with finesse. These sessions were like a breath of fresh air amidst the looming chaos, as everyone transformed into what we affectionately dubbed "Martians." Little did we realise then that this quirky dress code would soon become our new normal for the foreseeable future. Who knew we were trendsetters in intergalactic fashion?

There was daily mixed messaging and in a swift turn of events, we transitioned from assuring people that masks were unnecessary to suddenly mandating their use for everyone. But these weren't just any masks; we had upgraded to FFP3 masks, which required meticulous fit testing for each individual to guarantee maximum protection.

The testing took at least 20-30 minutes for each person, and that was if they passed the first time. If the masks did not fit their face then an alternative would need to be tested and ultimately a full headpiece needed to be used for those who failed on the commonly used available masks. I say available – this was yet another issue. The make of masks changed as stocks ran low and the threat of masks becoming unavailable was real. This was an enormous task, but we got through it.

Before long we realised we had more patients than our divided unit could cope with and this resulted in us converting even more wards into intensive care units, again not an easy task. How on earth were we going to look after all these patients?

All planned activity in the hospital came to a stop and nurses were deployed to work with us. I knew this was terrifying for them, as they had never worked in intensive care and most of the nurses were from theatres or recovery where their patient contact was very different.

While both theatre nursing and intensive care nursing involve caring for patients in the acute care settings, they differ in terms of focus, patient population and the level of acuity. Theatre nursing emphasises surgical care, while intensive care nursing focuses on the management of critically ill patients in a specialised intensive care setting.

Staff were nervous about coming to us; many expressed the concern that they had babies or young children. I was constantly asked if they would be safe to go home. All I could do at this point was support them and equip them with the best training possible.

We then had some staff with medical conditions of their own which meant they were unable to work in a Covid area. This posed a logistical nightmare. We had limited nurses trained in intensive care and had to spread them across four units, three Covid areas and one non-Covid, what we referred to as our green area. As of course, we still had sick non-Covid patients to look after.

A typical 'normal' busy shift in the Intensive Care Unit

often meant dealing with a tight staff-to-patient ratio, which could be especially challenging when admitting severely ill patients. Those who had been under our supervision for over 24 hours were usually stabilised, with their treatment progressing steadily. However, acute admissions often necessitated complex procedures like hemofiltration to support failing kidneys or post-operative monitoring following abdominal surgery or cardiac arrests. Additionally, almost every patient required a central line for administering medication and fluids efficiently.

The daily routine involved meticulous care of these lines and constant monitoring, adhering to strict protocols for dressing changes and documentation. Despite the demanding workload, the dedicated teamwork of the intensive care staff ensured that tasks were managed effectively, with each member supporting one another throughout the intense 12-hour shifts.

While physically and mentally exhausting, these challenging days were also deeply rewarding, and filled with a sense of accomplishment and pride in the team's achievements. However, the sense of control that characterised these shifts was notably absent during the pandemic. It felt like being on a roller coaster without any safety measures or ability to steer, as we navigated through uncertainty and external pressures, feeling powerless in the face of uncontrollable forces.

Three weeks into the pandemic, the country found itself gripped by an unprecedented crisis, with lockdown measures in full force. Within the confines of the intensive care unit, nurses, typically accustomed to a 1-1 patient ratio, were now stretched thin, grappling with ratios of 1-3 patients per nurse, or even 1-4. The toll of this strain was evident: nurses, weary and emotionally drained, found themselves leaving shifts in tears, their faces bearing the physical scars of prolonged mask wearing. Despite their best efforts, the weight of the situation bore down heavily on them. They soldiered on, performing admirably in the face of overwhelming odds, yet their own feelings of inadequacy and sorrow lingered. As the pandemic's grasp tightened, the intensity of the situation only escalated, each passing day bringing with it new challenges and uncertainties.

One day, not long into the chaos, I received a call from inside the unit. I was told that one of the nurses was struggling and could I go and help. I spoke with my consultant and we both donned our protective clothing before entering the unit. As we walked into the bustling area my phone started ringing from my pocket. I couldn't answer it as I was gowned up. It was persistent; it rang about five times, so I knew something must be wrong, someone needed me. My consultant agreed that I should leave the unit and answer the phone. He was happy to take over and deal with the situation on the unit.

I eventually answered the phone. It was the care home my dad was in and they proceeded to tell me that dad was very unwell and I should come to the home immediately. I did just that. I spoke to a colleague and phoned my manager from the car as I drove, with a sense of apprehension, to be with my dad.

The storm of the pandemic was more than a global crisis—it was a personal reckoning. As fear and uncertainty swirled around me, the lessons from my inner work became lifelines, grounding me amidst the chaos. I had spent so much time preparing for resilience, but was I truly ready for the reality of what was to come? The days ahead would stretch me in ways I had never imagined—mentally, physically, and emotionally. No amount of preparation could have fully equipped me for the relentless wave of suffering and heartbreak that awaited. As I stepped deeper into the fire, I knew one thing: I had to trust myself. But even lifelines can fray under pressure. In the next chapter, the collision of personal grief and professional duty forces me to confront heartbreak in its rawest form.

CHAPTER 6

Heartfelt Choices

On April 13th 2020, Easter Monday, I wrote a reflective piece from the previous few days in my journal. I was sitting in a care home, where my father had been a resident for the past 18 months. He had Alzheimer's, a torturous disease of the brain that slowly destroys memory and thinking skills and eventually takes away the ability to carry out the simplest of tasks.

Dad had been diagnosed at the age of 72. Mum and dad had retired to Ireland, their home country, but once dad had this diagnosis, they returned to the UK so mum could be supported by myself and my three sisters. Admitting dad to the care facility wasn't a simple choice, but it had become unsafe for him at home, and we felt compelled to make that decision.

I often ask myself, why didn't we look after dad at home? After all, there were four of us girls. Then I remember the countless incidents we had and the utter exhaustion on mum's face.

I recall an incident when I got a call from mum one night as dad had fallen in the bathroom. He was trapped behind the door and she wasn't able to help him. It took me and my partner to eventually prise the door open and help dad up on his feet. He had become quite unstable and the stairs were a big worry. His feet would barely be on the steps as he went up them.

One Tuesday afternoon at about 4 pm I got a call from mum saying dad had walked out of the house and she couldn't get him to come back inside. I didn't live very far away so I drove round as quickly as possible, thinking he would be just wandering around the cul-de-sac where they lived.

When I arrived, my sister was there walking alongside dad trying to persuade him to turn around and walk the other way. She had arrived for a visit having just finished work and walked in to find mum in a panic because dad had got out. Mum used to keep the doors locked, as this wasn't the first time. If you have had any experience with someone who has Alzheimer's you will know how determined they become.

My dad was a very quiet man, not surprising given the fact that he lived with a houseful of women. He had his routines and was never one for long conversations. Mum was the disciplinarian and housekeeper; dad went with the flow. I never heard my dad swear and he hardly ever raised his voice; if he did, it was usually for good reason. That was until his disease progressed. He was prone to quite violent outbursts, and it was difficult to calm him down.

I joined my sister as we both attempted to take dad's hand and guide him in a different direction. Unfortunately, instead of walking around the cul-de-sac, he was heading towards the road. When he got to the road he then continued towards a very busy dual carriageway and we knew we had to stop him, somehow. Deb decided she would run back to the house as we didn't have a phone between us. I'm not sure who she was going to call, but we needed help.

I continued with my dad on his unstoppable journey. We got to the dual carriageway and I had to physically get in his way to stop him from stepping straight into the busy rush hour traffic, a split-second decision that could have altered the course of our life. He was walking at a fast pace and wouldn't answer anything I said to him. His face was fixed and he was staring ahead with a look of determination. When I tried to hold his arm he just pushed me away and swore at me vehemently. It was terrifying. As cars thundered by, tears streamed down my face, and I was aiming frantic cries at my dad. I was desperate to shield him from the imminent danger looming ahead. We had now travelled a long way along the dual carriageway.

Suddenly a woman pulled over and asked if I needed help. Thank goodness for her. I very quickly explained the situation as the stranger seemed to stop dad in his tracks. She spoke to him and asked if he wanted to sit in her car as he must be tired. He agreed and we managed to get him home. It had been one of the most terrifying experiences I have ever had.

It was at this point that we knew we would have to consider alternative arrangements. We had asked for help from social services and the Alzheimer's Society but dad had totally refused to engage with any carers and had become quite aggressive towards them. This was taking its toll on all of us, but particularly Mum.

It was suggested that respite care might be a good idea. It would give Mum a break and give us time to make a plan. We looked at several care homes that offered such care. Eventually we found one that we thought would suit Dad well. It didn't have the smell of stale urine so often noticeable in many of these places, though it wasn't particularly 'posh'. We had looked at some that were like hotels but not like home, and they appeared to be more concerned about the way they looked rather than the residents. This place was comfortable and clean, and it had staff who were very honest about what sometimes happens, but also they seemed to care. They had all sorts of entertainment and gadgets for Alzheimer's sufferers to engage in. This home was about a 30-minute drive away, but we all drove so that was fine.

I can't even begin to explain how it felt the day dad went in. My mum and younger sister took him in with a few of his belongings to try and help him settle. His room was basic and mum had sewn his name into all his clothes, which they hung in the wardrobe. Once they left they were told not to visit for at least a week as dad would need to settle. That was a long week and not without its challenges, but he eventually settled and that respite care eventually turned into his home.

When I arrived at the home after being urgently called away from the unit, an unsettling quiet greeted me. I hurried straight to dad's room, where he lay in bed, his breathing shallow and his face unusually flushed. As I gently touched his arm, I felt the strange chill of his skin, a stark contrast to the warmth in his cheeks. He was difficult to rouse no matter how softly I spoke or how firmly I tried to wake him. My heart sank, a heavy sense of foreboding settling in as I recognised the gravity of his condition. With a mix of professional urgency and personal dread, I reached out to my family to update them on the situation, knowing that this was a moment we had all hoped not to face.

The doctor had been called and had prescribed antibiotics for a suspected chest infection. The home also requested a Covid test, which took place the next day. Dad stayed in this state, barely responsive, for a few days.

I have always felt that end of life care is important and in intensive care we pride ourselves on giving the best end of life possible. Never before had this been more evident to me than it was then, as highlighted by an extract from my journal on that day:

> Monday 13th April 20:35
> *My dad is struggling. He has had many chest infections over the past few years, and we have nearly lost him a few times, nothing like this though. I fear there is no going back this time. He hasn't eaten or drunk anything for four to five days now. His breathing is noisy, and he looks like he is struggling. I hope with all my heart he doesn't feel how he looks.*

The local GP had been contacted again and had tried to refer dad to the palliative care team so they could set up a syringe driver for pain relief. As it was a Bank Holiday, they had refused the referral, saying they had no capacity. Community nurses were also contacted, but the same applied. The doctor prescribed what he could to relieve pain, but to me it wasn't working. Dad still looked uncomfortable, in pain and distressed.

Dad now had a confirmed diagnosis of COVID-19, and with it came a decision that no family should ever have to face. We could stay with Dad, but it meant confining ourselves to his room 24/7, unable to leave or return once the door had closed behind us. Until now, his room had offered a small reprieve, with its direct access to the gardens, allowing us to step outside without navigating through the care home's main corridors, but the new guidance left no room for compromise.

The moment my mum and two of my sisters said their goodbyes will stay with me forever. They kissed him gently, their faces etched with sorrow, whispering words of love and gratitude through tear-streaked cheeks. Each step they took towards the door felt like a weight pulling them further into an unbearable reality—that they might never see him again. My sister Deb and I chose to stay, but as the door closed behind them, the finality of their departure hit me like a tidal wave. It wasn't just a goodbye; it was a heart-breaking acknowledgment of what we all feared was coming, a grief so profound it left the air thick with silence and despair.

The weight of guilt was crushing as I stood torn between staying by my dad's side and fulfilling my duties at work. I felt pulled in opposite directions, each choice loaded with its own heavy burden. On one hand, the urge to be there for my dad in his final moments was overpowering, yet on the other, the knowledge that my skills and presence were desperately needed elsewhere was equally undeniable.

In that moment of turmoil, I grappled with the realisation that guilt, no matter how consuming, would serve no purpose for anyone involved. It would not ease my dad's suffering, nor could it alleviate the strain on the healthcare system. Instead, it threatened to paralyse me, rendering me incapable of offering genuine support on either hand.

Amidst the chaos, I clung to the principles of compassion and understanding. I reminded myself that while I couldn't be in two places at once, I could offer my presence and care in the moments I could spare, both to my dad and to my colleagues in the ITU. I sought solace in the knowledge that by honouring these principles, I could navigate through the storm of guilt and find a semblance of peace amidst the turmoil.

We have the power of choice over what we think. I knew what I was thinking, but did I know what I was feeling? Were my heart and mind in alignment?

At that time I was caught in a whirlwind of thoughts and responsibilities, constantly moving from one task to the next without pausing to truly reflect on my feelings. I was so preoccupied with the mental noise and the urgent demands of the situation that I failed to connect with what my heart was telling me. This lack of alignment between my thoughts and emotions left me feeling unsettled and burdened by guilt. It was only in retrospect, after having taken the time to reflect and gain perspective, that I found the clarity and peace I needed. I realised that my actions, driven by a flurry of thoughts rather than a true sense of inner understanding, were not fully in harmony with my deeper values and emotions. This process of reflection allowed me to reconcile with the decisions I had made and come to terms with the emotional turmoil I had been experiencing.

However, at the time I was far from at peace. I was questioning my every move and whether I was doing enough.

In the fragile space between life and death, the heart often speaks louder than logic. The choices I faced were steeped in love, guilt, and an aching sense of responsibility, blurring the lines between daughter and nurse. Each moment demanded a decision, but no answer ever felt wholly right. I had to navigate the impossible showing up for dad while knowing that my absence was felt elsewhere. Could I truly be present in both spaces at once? Or would my heart always carry the weight of what I had to leave behind? As I move forward, grief becomes both a companion and a teacher, shaping how I find meaning beyond loss in the chapters ahead.

CHAPTER 7

The Shadow of Sorrow

The nights in the nursing home were horrendous. The nurses' response time to our call bell was approximately one and a half hours when I would have expected it to be less than five minutes.

Even if staff cannot resolve an issue, it is still essential in these environments to acknowledge the patient as soon as possible, to ensure it is not truly urgent and everyone is safe. In the morning, after many discussions with the manager, it was agreed that dad would have regular four-hourly pain relief with top up when required.

It wasn't easy for the care home. They too had many challenges with staff sickness and agency nurses filling in when they could get them. These nurses were not familiar with the patients, and many of the patients were sick. The staff were getting by the best they could, just like everyone else.

The next night came, and the nurses just didn't understand. They managed to make me feel like I was doing something wrong by requesting more medication, and I began questioning myself. They would come and look at dad and say he was ok, no monitoring, no heart rate, no oxygen levels and no respiratory rate monitored. It was an extremely distressing night.

Monday 13th April 20:35
I am an intensive care nurse, why can I not look after my own dad? I would never let anyone end their life in this way and here I am watching my dad struggle with absolutely no ability to help him, why is no one helping us? In the morning my sister and I gave dad a good wash and splashed on his old spice, his favourite aftershave. He looked a little better and smelt wonderful, but his extremities were starting to look blue and mottled.

Wednesday 15th April 09:52
What a night. At approximately 6pm dad took yet another turn for the worse, how was this even possible? This time his breathing became silent, it was shallow and slow. Is this it, I thought to myself? His body was cold, his legs more mottled, we thought this was the end. We phoned my sisters, who were with my mum, and started to play dad's favourite music. I sat stroking dad's hands whilst Deb rubbed his forehead. We talked to him, reas-

suring him that everything would be ok, we would look after mum and each other. We told him what a fantastic dad he had been and how he had always been our stable, our rock. Dad kept going, occasionally taking a deep breath but his pulse was strong, his heart was strong. At about 2100hrs dad went back to breathing as he had been over the past few days. He wasn't ready to go.

On Thursday morning, we washed dad as usual and he smelt delicious, but his breathing was unpredictable from one minute to the next. A nurse came in and brought an oximeter with her. Dad's oxygen level was 64% and his heart rate was 130bpm. Both parameters were well outside normal. He became noticeably uncomfortable again, so we asked for more pain relief.

The GP was doing a virtual review of dad and we were asked to step into the garden area. I refused as we were the ones who had spent every minute with dad and were therefore best placed to answer questions. The review continued, but I had to intervene when the nurse answering the doctor stuttered and stumbled with the answers; it didn't feel like the important information was being clearly communicated. The doctor said dad looked very comfortable and used some other bland words; it all felt very vague and dismissive.

He then asked me a question, at which point unfortunately all my anger and frustration that had been building inside came out as I proceeded to tell him and the nurse exactly what I thought of the lack of care my dad had received. I did raise my voice and it wasn't my finest hour, but my sister stepped in to calm the situation down. I sobbed uncontrollably into my dad's chest as the devastation of what was happening took over.

About an hour later dad started coughing, choking and drowning in his own secretions. We called for help and once again it was slow in coming. When they did arrive I demanded some suction, in order to remove the secretions from dad's mouth and airways, which they eventually brought.

After watching my dad struggle for some time, the manager made the decision to call an ambulance urgently. This marked a significant change, as we had all previously agreed to avoid a hospital admission, believing they caused more harm than good. But this situation was different—something had shifted, and the need for immediate medical intervention was undeniable.

When the crew arrived, they asked questions about dad: where was his syringe driver, his medication, his care plan? We looked at the paramedics with tears running down our faces and just said 'exactly'. They were like angels sent from heaven.

Dad was bubbling like a boiling kettle; I have never heard anything like this in all my career of nursing. I used to be a specialist nurse for organ donation and never have I witnessed such poor palliative care. The paramedics administered morphine and spoke to the GP. They managed to get him to prescribe regular morphine and more glycopyrrolate, which helps dry secretions, then proceeded to go to the chemist and get the prescription themselves.

Courtney was one of the young paramedics. I'm convinced she was an angel, with tied-back blonde hair and a soft, gentle complexion. She asked us if we would consider sending dad to a hospice. We agreed immediately – he needed more help. After a short period of time, they had the hospice on the phone, and they asked to speak to me. They explained that from what they had been told he might not make the journey, despite it being only four miles away. I acknowledged this risk but said we would be prepared to take it, we just had to get out. Within 30 minutes we had packed dad up and left the home – it felt like we had kidnapped him. We didn't say goodbye, have a discussion or look back, just a swift exit. Deb went in the ambulance, and I followed.

When we arrived, I had no idea if dad was still going to be with us. My heart was racing, my palms sweating, and I felt nauseous. The doors opened and there were dad and Deb listening to Neil Diamond. We were greeted at the door by a lovely nurse and escorted inside. Deb and I were put into a waiting room while they settled dad.

The doctor came in to speak to us. She looked quite distressed herself with what appeared to be tears in her eyes. She didn't know dad, but the state he was in was clearly too much for anyone to witness. She explained that they would get the syringe driver set up and give dad enough medication to keep him comfortable. They decided that given the fact we had been with dad every day, we could now stay with him. This was despite having been told previously that we would only be able to stay an hour. They were so compassionate and caring; we were very grateful.

We went in to be with dad, and he looked very comfortable, more so than he had been for the past week. The duvet was blue, crisp and clean with ironed sheets. The room was clean and tidy, and dad looked really peaceful. He had been accustomed to this type of sheet and bedding, as mum was very fastidious. They brought a reclining chair that Deb slept in, though I use the word 'slept' loosely. I sat beside dad with my legs up on a chair, one eye open and ears pricked.

At approximately 3 am we noticed a change in dad's breathing. He inhaled and exhaled slowly with the time between breaths becoming longer and longer.

At 0430, he took his last breath.

Saturday 18th April 13:05
Dad passed away Friday 17th April 04:30 at The Hos-

pice. How did this happen? Quite simply the worst week and the worst experience of my life.

We felt mixed emotions; relief, but also deep sorrow. Dad had clearly not wanted to die at the care home. Deb had always struggled with the memories of taking dad in there with my mum, but at least now she had also had the chance to take him out to somewhere like home, somewhere peaceful and comforting. The sheets and blankets he lay in enveloped him like he was receiving a huge hug, clearly what he needed and where he needed to be before he had let go.

Even though you may be aware and have time to 'prepare' yourself before someone dies, nothing really prepares you, and I was left feeling numb.

Watching my father struggle without the proper care he deserved was a nightmare I wouldn't wish on anyone. These were nights that tested my faith in the systems I had once trusted implicitly and forced me to confront the stark realities of healthcare in crisis. But this chapter was not the end—it was merely a turning point. The following pages explore how these experiences pushed me further into my own journey of grief, resilience, and, ultimately, healing; underlining that it is often darkest before the dawn.

CHAPTER 8

Resilience and loss

The unit continued to be an enormous worry. I had just left one day and not returned for what was now three weeks, as I had had to self-isolate after dad had gone. These were the rules put in place to try and help stop or at least slow the virus.

The day before I was due to return to work, my dog, my beautiful golden retriever Izzy, became unwell. She had been with me since she was eight weeks old and was now 14. She had been struggling to get around and on this morning she collapsed to the ground a few times with sad eyes that were drooping and tired.

I took her to the emergency vet, who suspected that she had suffered a stroke. This, along with her incontinence and lack of mobility, led us to the very tough decision to put her to sleep later that day.

We took her home and I called the children, who

came to say a heart-wrenching goodbye. She just lay with her tail wagging as she was kissed and cuddled. Another tough decision: was I doing the right thing, was this really her time to go? I chatted with my sister and came to the realisation that despite Izzy's ability to continue to respond, she was struggling.

Initially the vet had said that due to the Covid rules I would need to just leave her, but this was never going to happen; I would rather keep her by my side and wait until things changed. Luckily the vet could see this and acknowledged that I was going to stay with her. She suggested attaching an extended line to administer the drugs that would lay her to rest.

Izzy lay on my lap and I cuddled her, giving her all the love I could in my arms as she closed her eyes for the final time. She was my true companion, the one stable thing in my life, always loving me no matter what happened. I was already feeling that my heart was broken but now, I felt it had been ripped out of me. I was exhausted, depleted of all my energy and once again left with overwhelming sadness.

I remember looking up towards the heavens, hands open with my arms out and shouting 'What the fuck! Why?'

When I returned to work, I went back onto autopilot. Rotas, staffing, sick patients, staff in crisis – it really is all a blur. I do remember during some downtime wondering how I was going to get through this, how we were all going to get through it.

I discussed what was happening with a dear friend who lives in France and who I had become close to during our personal development journey. She suggested I do an exercise we had been taught in a lesson called 'Mastering Emotions'. This exercise involved asking myself several questions and keeping going with the answers until I had exhausted all possibilities in my mind. I sat and duly did as she suggested.

When I first began working through this exercise, I found myself facing questions that required an uncomfortable level of honesty and introspection. These questions weren't designed to provide quick answers; instead, they served as a pathway to uncover deeper truths hidden beneath layers of emotion and assumptions. Each question was a step toward clarity, growth, and, ultimately, transformation.

The first question, "What actually happened?", demands a detachment from the emotional narrative we often attach to events. By focusing solely on the facts, this question helps strip away the fog of our emotions, biases, and judgments. It's not about what I felt or perceived but about identifying the raw, unaltered truth of the situation. For me, this meant acknowledging, without dramatising, that my dad had passed away. This simple, unembellished fact became the foundation upon which the rest of the exercise would build.

The second question, "What does that mean?", took me one layer deeper. Here, the goal is to examine the significance we assign to an event. This is where emotions can subtly creep back in, so it was important to approach this step with a clear and conscious mind. For me, it meant recognising that I would no longer see my father in the physical world. Stripped of the emotional weight, this truth created space for acceptance and understanding.

The third question, "What can I learn from this event?", is where the heart of the exercise lies. It encourages a shift from victimhood to empowerment, asking me to search for the lessons hidden within my pain. It's not always easy or immediate, but the act of seeking meaning allows us to transform even the most challenging experiences into valuable insights. This question reminded me that within every hardship lies an opportunity for growth—if I was willing to search for it.

Finally, "I am grateful for this happening because..." pushed me to the edge of my comfort zone. Gratitude, especially in the face of loss, can feel impossible at first. But when we dig deep, listing at least ten reasons we're grateful for the event, we begin to uncover hidden gifts. Perhaps it brought me closer to the rest of my family, or it deepened my compassion for others experiencing grief. Each reason became a piece of treasure, helping me reframe the narrative of the event in a way that brings peace and closure.

The true magic of this exercise lies in persistence. It's not about stopping when you find one or two answers—it's about exhausting every possibility until the gifts are undeniable. When you can look at the event and recognise its value without bitterness or regret, you've dug deep enough to uncover the treasure within. At that moment, the event is no longer a source of pain but a catalyst for transformation.

With everything going on right now there were many things I could have focused on, so I chose what was most intense for me at that moment, dad passing away.

I used this exercise to move from emotional suffering to peace. The key results of this, i.e. the new perspectives I was able to attain, were:

If my dad had not become unwell with Alzheimer's he might never have come back to the UK. He might have died at some point for some reason in Ireland and there was a possibility I would not have been there to hold his hand, to have months of sitting with him reminiscing about our childhood holidays in Wales and Cornwall. Our holidays were always fun, and we had many magic moments to remember.

Though our adventures were often filled with laughter and joy, there's one memory that stands out, etched into my mind with a mix of affection and sheer terror.

We were in Cornwall, playing on the beach, when Dad, ever the adventurous spirit, led us towards the edge of the sea. With his firm grasp holding mine and my sister's hands, we felt safe and secure. Yet, in an instant, a monstrous wave crashed over us, engulfing our senses in a noise of bubbling water. Panic overwhelmed me as I struggled to orientate myself in the chaos, fearing the worst. But through it all, Dad held onto us tightly, ensuring we were safe. To this day, I can't help but shudder at the thought of submerging my head underwater, a lingering reminder of that heart-stopping incident on the shore.

Dad was pivotal in our family and coming back to the UK meant we all became much closer again. We hadn't drifted apart due to a lack of love for each other, just because life has a way of allowing you to drift as you get caught up in your own day-to-day life.

I was now able to see that I had been given an opportunity. I was grateful that dad never had to suffer the loss of one of his children. Throughout the evolution of life there has been a fundamental expectation deeply ingrained in the fabric of existence: the idea that parents will precede their children in death. This expectation is rooted in the natural order of life, where parents typically provide guidance, protection, and support to their offspring, nurturing them as they grow and develop. However, in the modern human experience, this expectation has been profoundly challenged by advances in medicine, technology, and societal norms. With improved healthcare and living conditions, the average lifespan has increased significantly, leading to a paradigm shift where parents now anticipate seeing their children grow into adulthood and beyond. Yet, despite these advancements, the inherent fragility and unpredictability of life remain, serving as a poignant reminder that the expectation of parents outliving their children is not always guaranteed.

This realisation underscores the preciousness of every moment we share with our loved ones and the importance of cherishing the time we have together, for life's journey is as unpredictable as it is precious.

I realised there is no certainty in life, and this sequence of events had opened my eyes to what I really want from the school of life I am currently in. What I now realise is that everything does happen for a reason but sometimes you need to dig deep and do the work to find it. Sometimes, the profound gifts hidden within life's events are shrouded in layers of emotion. The intensity of these reactions can obscure our ability to perceive the underlying blessings. It's in those moments of deep emotional turbulence that the task of unravelling these layers becomes especially challenging, yet it is often through this process of digging deep, confronting our emotions and doing the inner work that we can begin to uncover the valuable insights and gifts that lie beneath the surface.

This is when I came to realise the true power of the mind. I went from feeling beaten, battered and destroyed to being utterly grateful for the events that had taken place.

Thank goodness for the time and energy I had previously invested into my self-development work. Although I had not continued with all of my practices while I was with dad, I had continued to journal, which was an emotional lifeline for me.

> *Resilience is not built in moments of ease, but in the depths of loss and uncertainty. As I reflect on the heartbreak of saying goodbye to Izzy and dad, I see how grief can hollow you out, yet also carve space for a deeper understanding of love, connection, and the impermanence of life. The pain felt unbearable, but through self-inquiry and perspective shifts, I found hidden gifts in these moments—treasures of gratitude, clarity, and strength that I never expected. Loss is inevitable, but how we choose to navigate it defines our healing. In the next chapter, I continue this journey, exploring the profound ways in which hardship can shape and transform us.*

CHAPTER 9

Finding Strength Through Reflection

I am still in awe at how incredible the staff on our ITU were. Their job is busy and difficult at the best of times, but now they were also having to carry the concern that they might take the virus home, so many of them were fearing for the safety of their families as well as their patients. On top of this, every news outlet was talking as if this was the end of life as we know it. What a situation!

The physical strength it took to come in day after day, with dressings over the bridges of our noses to help prevent further sores developing, alongside the mental turmoil, was beyond demanding. I know many drove home in tears as they were left feeling exhausted, stripped of all their energy and goodwill.

I wonder now if the personal development work I had started would have helped everyone, not just the doctors and nurses but everyone else; porters, cleaners, care assistants, canteen staff; I wonder how much suffering could have been avoided, both during and after this madness.

> *Would they have been able to process the events in a different way?*
>
> *Have they now locked the trauma away, burying it deep inside?*
>
> *How long can this trauma remain buried before it begins to negatively affect them?*
>
> *Would this all manifest in the future as a positive or negative reality?*
>
> *Would they be able to remember, with pride, the courage each and every one of them had shown?*

I unknowingly used many different tools for processing my thoughts and feelings during the intensity of the pandemic, one of which was writing, hence this book.

The following is a poem I wrote in the early hours of one morning whilst I was humbly reflecting on the day gone by. I'm not a poet, but I have always dabbled with diaries, and as this was such a deep emotional challenge we faced, it felt natural to return to writing.

I just wrote and wrote from my heart, a bit like a runner who just keeps going and going until there is nothing left.

In the Shadows of Care

The unit phone rings, it's answered with care
Outreach on the line, is a doctor there?
We have a patient in need of your care.

The nurses act fast, the doctors with speed
The bed space is checked and has everything we need.

Bang goes the door, no time to veer
In rolls the patient, a herd draws near
The doctors and nurses are all masked up
Gowns, gloves and visors, someone has to speak up.
The patient looks scared, her eyes tell a tale
Her SATS start to drop and she looks very pale

Her skin is clammy, her face looks marked
She's had a tight-fitting mask and looks visibly scarred.
We welcome her kindly, there are people everywhere
She can barely speak now and just looks with a stare.

We tell her it's time for the tight-fitting mask,
We know what it's like, we feel guilty to ask.
Some say it's like putting your head out of the car,
It's difficult to breathe due to the force and the gasp.
She has some sedation, this helps her to cope
We settle her quickly and can only hope.

CHRISTINE REDMOND

The bloods are taken, the observations recorded
It's obvious now this should be aborted.
The doctor talks slowly, in a calm, peaceful voice,
Muffled, he sweetly outlines our choice.
He tells her it's the end of this tight-fitting mask
And in order to save her we must act fast.

As she moves into sleep, our steps become clear,
While this is intense, it's why we are here.
The tube is in place which supports her to breath,
We want her to stay, it's not her time to leave.
We're on the right path, it's all going well,
When suddenly we lose output, not this again, oh hell!

Resuscitation starts with a nurse pressing hard,
On her chest that needs pressure for her heart to restart.
Drugs are given timely, and we continue our task,
One hour to save a life that could easily pass.

Her body looks grey, purple and blue,
There is no hope now, everyone knew.
At one hour in, the doctor calls time,
Does everyone agree? This is such a crime.
We stop with great sadness, sorrow in our hearts,
Silence surrounds us, as another departs.

The doctor calls the family, the fourth of the day
An exasperating experience, why is it this way?
The nurses prepare her with love and with care
Washing and cleaning her for viewing, we are there.
The family attend with grief and in pain,
We all stand around, feeling the same.

Why does this keep happening?
It's cruel and unfair
There needs to be an end
There needs to be a prayer.

The staff leave the unit, broken and sad,
Knowing tomorrow will also be bad.

It's a difficult time, but hope is not lost.
They are the light in the darkness
Providing hope amongst fear
A connection for families,
To pass on love to ones so dear.

We can't always cure patients,
We've lost too many to count.
This is not what we are used to,
Not this amount.

As with all things, this challenge did pass.
Although at the time, it did not leave fast.

They come back to see us,
we celebrate success.
Nursed back from illness,
smiling at their best.

As I re-read these lines, I am reminded of the persistent hope that guides us through these trying times.

Have you ever tried writing non-stop for a minimum of five minutes? We call it the 'hot pen exercise'. Reflect on an area of your life you would like to change, and in relation to that ask yourself a question you do not know the answer to. Then simply write, without filter, whatever comes up. It may be a lot, it may be a little, there is no right or wrong. This is an exercise of inner inquiry, and therefore whatever comes up can be considered a gift of greater awareness. You will be surprised how it feels when you're finished.

> *Grief carves deep, hollow spaces within us, but it also makes room for growth we never expected. Through reflection, I began to see the threads of resilience woven into even the darkest moments. The pain I had endured, the losses I had faced—they were not just burdens to carry, but stepping stones toward a deeper*

understanding of who I was becoming. This realisation shifted something within me. No longer was I simply surviving; I was rebuilding, reimagining what my life could be. In the next chapter, I embrace the lessons of these reflections, stepping into a future defined not by what I've lost, but by how I've chosen to rise.

CHAPTER 10

Embracing the Future

I had just finished the Elite Mentorship Forum, a six-month programme aimed at overcoming personal and worldly limiting beliefs. Finally I was starting to feel just a little better, even though I was fully aware it was early days and I had more work to do.

I now felt called to complete the coach training I had started back in 2019. I remember it clearly. I had gone on holiday with my family. It was when the world had opened up for a brief moment in time. We were in Cyprus, and I dedicated the first two to three hours of every sunny, warm morning sitting by the pool. I would be committed to this training. Finally, in October 2020, I had completed all the modules and assignments and had the certificate a few weeks later to confirm passing the course. A good example of an achievement that felt great for about half a day. This was still just the beginning of my journey.

As time progressed and despite the continued effects of the pandemic, I came to a firm realisation: it was imperative that I take decisive action, summon my courage, and refuse to allow fear to hinder my progress. In February 2021, I took a definitive step forward by enrolling as one of the inaugural trainers for Peter Sage.

To be a trainer really resonated with me. I would be helping people who needed what I could give, synergising my nursing and my Tony Robbins training, and I would be able to guide people through the same proven transformational process which had been so valuable for me.

I consciously shifted my focus away from concerns about financial stability and uncertainty, and instead embraced a path where I was confident in my ability to succeed and positively impact others. It marked a new chapter in my journey—a commitment to giving back and making a meaningful contribution to those around me.

If life were like a fairytale, then this realisation would be the turning point at which I could begin to live my dreams, but life is far more tortuous and has rapids and waterfalls that make it more of a wild torrent than a smoothly-flowing river. At no time was this more viscerally obvious to me than when I was faced with the prospect of my own mortality, the fear that my heart had stopped doing what it should, and it was possibly time for me to leave this life.

Upon returning from my break, I thought things were starting to get a little better. In August 2020 the government had introduced a scheme called 'Eat Out to help Out', encouraging people to return to normal living. Then later that month rules were relaxed further as indoor theatres, bowling alleys and soft play areas were reopened. However, the media once again started reporting negative news and many people were in a state of panic about their own mortality or their businesses. Many hospitality venues had struggled through the first lockdown and despite the schemes in place, some were on the brink of bankruptcy.

Daily news reports once again spoke of the rising number of deaths. We heard from publicans, restaurateurs, nightclub owners etc stressing caution about us being plunged into another lockdown, for fear of the consequences this would have on the economy.

Then, once again, it happened. Within weeks, on 31st October 2020, we were hit with a second wave and a new lockdown.

Even though we had become adept at caring for these patients, my heart sank as we found ourselves in a worse position with many more people dying. We had learnt a lot in the first wave, but somehow this didn't seem to help. Once again staff were deployed to us, even doctors that are rarely seen at the bedside to give patient care.

The pressures mounted again, and I regularly asked myself how this was even possible.

My role during the pandemic was significantly different from that which I'd fulfilled during the rest of my career. Now each day I was faced with the same issues:

> *"Green area, Red area 1, 2 or 3?"*
> *"Have the ventilators been counted this morning?"*
> *"How many pumps are in use?"*
> *"Has the equipment audit been carried out?"*
> *"How many patients are we expecting?"*
> *"How many beds can we staff?"*
> *"What does the rest of the region look like?"*
> *"Do I have all the figures for the first of our many daily calls?"*
> *"How is my newly created battle board looking?"*

Yes, I really was in an episode of MASH!

Were we going to have a full-on war today? Or perhaps we would be blessed with a short ceasefire.

> 5th January 2021 22:35
>
> *What a week, the pandemic has hit ridiculous levels again. Tempers and emotions have been very high all week. I'm exhausted, tearful and tense.*
>
> *I sent a positive email to the bosses today. It had a positive vibe around staffing as I was very pleased to confirm we could staff and open 25 level 3 beds. The night shifts were still a bit low but I am confident we*

will get them covered. Unfortunately this email was not received in the spirit with which it had been sent. I had replies telling me this was not good enough and we needed a minimum of 26 level 3 beds open. This was very frustrating as what they didn't understand was that I was unlikely to have 26 level 3 patients at any one point. (Level 3 are fully ventilated dependent patients and require 1-1 nursing). We would have 26 beds open as level 1 & 2 don't require the same ratio and therefore the varying levels made 26 possible. The day continued in the same vein as I was told the chief executive was insisting on 26 beds. I tried to explain the scenario, but it just didn't seem to land. This was such a disappointment and quite frankly felt like a kick in the teeth as we had worked so hard to get to these levels. It wasn't just about the number of beds, it was about the care we could provide, looking out for staff and being realistic.

We had a good plan in ITU for a potential next wave and had run a mini course (teaching the basics of ITU) for several staff, picked out from various departments from around the hospital. Unfortunately, these staff were not the ones released once the second wave hit and therefore the tension and frustration was palpable.

I haven't been able to put into practice the high performance habits I had been learning. I have taken comments personally but that's because I care and feel passionate about doing the right thing for both staff and patients.

I could go on about what should have happened, but there is no point. We need to move forward as best we can and get as many people looked after properly as we can.

A few days later, it happened. I felt a funny feeling in my chest, and my heart was pounding. I placed my hand over it to try and slow the banging drum inside me. It didn't stop. I wasn't sweating, I wasn't dizzy, it didn't radiate down either of my arms or into my neck. I sat in this condition for about a minute until I heard the outer door to my office open.

The outreach team, who can best be described as a mobile intensive care unit, sat just outside my office. They had the unenviable task of providing a service to the whole of the hospital, going out seeing patients on the wards. They did such a good job, particularly during Covid, as they saw people early and implemented plans to try and prevent further deterioration and ultimate admission to the unit.

No sooner had they sat in their seats than I heard another alarm, the pager buzzing as its high-pitched sound summoned the nurses yet again. I knew they had barely been in their office all day, so I opened my door to check they were OK and find out what the situation was around the hospital.

Are we to expect more admissions?

How are the patients on the respiratory ward?

Do they have enough non-invasive ventilation machines for the number of patients needing them?

Are they ok?

I was given a brief update as Sarah, one of the nurses working with the outreach team, took a quick sip of water before she had to leave again.

"Oh, by the way, just so you know, I have a pain in my chest, if you come back and find me collapsed you know why!" I said this casually to Sarah with a hint of humour in my tone, yet underneath, a flicker of concern lingered. Despite my laughter, I couldn't shake off the gnawing sensation of discomfort. When Sarah raised an eyebrow and questioned me, I brushed it off with a smile and insisted I was okay, but the unease remained.

There is a saying: 'If you don't make time for your health, you'll have to make time for illness.' It's a warning I've heard before, but never truly absorbed. At the time, I felt invincible—I wasn't incapacitated, I wasn't bedridden with sickness; it was just a nagging discomfort. I briefly entertained the notion that it could be stress or anxiety, but quickly brushed it aside. After all, I had become used to the stress of the past year's pandemic and my mind wasn't any more weighed down with the burdens of stress than I had become used to.

Stress, to me, was a tangible sensation; it was a feeling that my head was on the brink of bursting, my body weighed down by an invisible force, and an overwhelming sense of directionlessness. But that's not what I thought I was experiencing. I was simply going about my day, quietly attending to the logistics of staff and patient ratios for the upcoming shifts. And so the day continued. I continued!

Over the following few months the pain came and went, varying in intensity, and I would stick my head out of the door to anyone who was around and just say 'girls, I have that pain again, just so you know'. It became laughable. That was until I had a few days off, when things had settled slightly and were going in the right direction in terms of the pandemic. I remember having four days at home just pottering and catching up on life. There it was again, that pain, that feeling. I had no one around to tell, no girls to shout across to and I wasn't at work so why did I have this pain again?

I was alone and this became even more evident. I like my own company and I have a large family that keep me busy, but, when something like this happens, that 'alone' feeling becomes magnified.

Should I ring and tell someone, would I be found dead in my house at some point?

Who would find me?

How awful was that going to be for someone to find me dead?

Thoughts like this kept swirling around in my head

until I eventually managed to tell myself I was being ridiculous.

Monkey chatter, which is what I call those tens of thousands of thoughts we have per day, can be dangerous. They range from fleeting and subconscious thoughts to more deliberate and focused ones. The mind is often active, and thoughts can arise from various stimuli, experiences, and internal processes. I have come to realise that they are not always true. Just because you think something, it doesn't make it real. To this day I must remind myself of this and ask myself different questions to eliminate those unwanted terrifying thoughts. I brought myself back into reality and rationalised that monkey chatter.

The following day I went about my business as usual. I chatted with one of our cardiac nurses who had been redeployed to work with us. I told her about my chest pains, which had now been going on for a few months, and she immediately went into full-on nurse consultant mode. Before I knew it, I had an ECG (Electrocardiogram, a recording of the heart's electrical activity). I was booked for an appointment with the cardiologist and bloods were drawn to check what was happening and if there were any abnormalities. On the day of the appointment with the cardiologist, I remember walking from the car park to the hospital, just a couple of hundred yards. My watch buzzed and when I looked at it, there it was: a heart rate of 170bpm. The average heart rate is between 65-75bpm, so I was double where I should be.

"Wow, I'm unfit", I thought as the pain started to creep back into my chest. Physical fitness is dynamic and multifaceted. I knew that common signs and symptoms include low cardiovascular endurance, shortness of breath, increased heart rate on exertion, fatigue and exhaustion, along with low mood and poor sleep, to name just a few. I was feeling all these things. When I looked back at the readings my watch had recorded over the past few weeks, I could see I had many peaks in my heart rate beyond what we would consider as normal, I was tired and I wasn't sleeping well.

Am I unfit?

Is fitness just physical?

No, we need to also look after our mental fitness.

Do we see a healthy person as someone who is physically fit, whose body is functioning as it should?

Are we as healthcare professionals fixated on the physical in isolation of someone's mental and emotional health?

Health encompasses a person's physical, mental and emotional state.

There have been huge advances in physical healthcare, but can the same be said for mental and emotional health?

The latest research shows that there has been a growing awareness of mental health issues globally, leading to increased recognition and discussion of mental health concerns. This has resulted in more people seeking the help they require. However, we can see disparities in access to mental health services continue to exist, with some communities often facing greater barriers to care. Issues such as availability of services, and cultural factors can influence access to essential support.

As healthcare professionals we can see in ourselves:

- Increased stress and burnout. Healthcare workers often face high levels of stress and burnout due to the demanding nature of their work, long hours, and exposure to trauma and suffering. The COVID-19 pandemic has intensified these stressors, with healthcare workers facing unprecedented challenges such as overwhelming patient loads, personal protective equipment (PPE) shortages, and fear of contracting the virus.

- Mental health disorders. Healthcare workers are at risk of developing mental health disorders such as anxiety, depression, post-traumatic stress disorder (PTSD), and substance abuse disorders. The demanding and emotionally taxing nature of their work, coupled with factors like stigma surrounding mental illness and reluctance to seek help, can contribute to the development of these disorders.

- **Emotional challenges.** Healthcare professionals often face significant emotional challenges as they navigate the complexities of their roles. Constant exposure to illness, suffering, and loss can take a toll on their emotional well-being, leading to feelings of compassion fatigue, burnout, and moral distress. They may grapple with the emotional weight of making life-altering decisions, witnessing patients' pain, and coping with their own limitations in providing care. Additionally, the demanding nature of their work, coupled with long hours and high-pressure environments, can contribute to stress, anxiety, and emotional exhaustion.

- **Work-life balance.** Maintaining a healthy work-life balance can be challenging for healthcare workers, especially during times of crisis. Long hours, irregular shifts and emotional strain can impact personal relationships, leisure activities, and overall well-being.

- **Support and resources.** Access to adequate support and resources is essential for promoting the good overall health of healthcare workers. This includes access to services such as peer support programs, counselling, and initiatives to promote self-care and resilience.

- Organisational culture: The culture within healthcare organisations plays a crucial role in supporting the overall health of workers. Cultures that prioritise employee well-being, provide opportunities for professional development, and foster open communication can help mitigate stress and burnout among healthcare staff.

- Recognition and appreciation. Recognising the efforts of healthcare workers and expressing appreciation for their contributions can have a positive impact on their health. Feeling valued and supported by colleagues, supervisors, and the broader community can help mitigate the negative effects of stress and burnout. We saw this happen during the pandemic as people clapped and cheered for healthcare professionals. But, what about now, are we truly appreciated?

Addressing the health needs of healthcare workers is critical for ensuring the well-being of those who care for others. Efforts to support the health & wellbeing of these key workers should be comprehensive, addressing both individual and systemic factors that contribute to stress and burnout in the healthcare setting.

Rant over. Back to my appointment.

When I eventually arrived, I had an ECHO (echocardiogram, an ultrasound scan of the heart) and the consultant reviewed all the tests. He found I had some ectopics, which are small disturbances of the heart but nothing outside what you would expect for a normal healthy person. However, I showed the doctor my heart rate readings and it was a concern. He decided to prescribe beta blockers for a few months and I was told to keep monitoring the episodes. These drugs block the stress response of adrenaline and noradrenaline.

My condition could only be put down to stress. I was a little confused. I wasn't necessarily getting these pains in those moments of feeling overwhelmed and anxious, the stress response I had come to know so well. I was feeling ok, a bit tired, still a little worried, but all in all I was ok.

I knew this was a warning. I had learned that life gives us warnings; they start as a little nudge, then a harder slap until eventually we get struck with what can feel like a sledgehammer until we take notice. I hadn't been taking time to relax properly. I would have a day off and be constantly looking at my phone or emails or answering calls about work. It was like a light bulb was constantly shining and only being slightly dimmed but never turned off.

Life has a way of nudging us, whispering when we need to listen, and shouting when we ignore the signs. My journey through resilience, loss, and the relentless demands of the pandemic had brought me here—to a moment where my own health forced me to pause and reflect. The body keeps score, and mine was sounding the alarm. But beyond the stress, beyond the exhaustion, was an opportunity: to recalibrate, to redefine what true well-being means—not just for myself, but for all those who dedicate their lives to helping others. In the next chapter, I explore what it truly means to slow down, be present, and reclaim a sense of purpose—not through doing more, but through learning the power of stillness, awareness, and deep, intentional rest.

CHAPTER 11

Reclaiming Purpose

How do we take the time to relax properly when there is so much to do? What does that even look like?

I realised that I was not finding *true* relaxation time. As I inquired into this, I uncovered something amazing; if we are not truly present in the moment, we can never truly relax. I was receiving those nudges but hadn't been noticing them.

My daughter had a baby in May 2020, my second grandson and a pure bundle of joy. She had a tough time having a first baby in lockdown, as I imagine many did. The disappearance of mother and baby groups meant there was very little support from other mums in the same situation.

My grandchildren bring about feelings that are hard to describe. When someone is pregnant, they will often ask, 'How do you know when you are in labour?' The response, 'You will know' is all anyone can truly say, as it's an experience that is like nothing else. Also, if you told them what it's really like they would be utterly terrified. Anyway, the overwhelming love I feel for my grandchildren is like that. It's the most magical feeling of unconditional love that I have ever felt and is difficult to describe.

Despite this love, I had one of those nudges in May 2022. The pandemic had settled for the outside world and was finally settling within the hospital. I was taking my grandson for a walk along the river. It was a sunny day, there were blossom on the trees and just a slight chill in the air which made it fresh and invigorating. We fed the ducks, talked about all the swans and generally chatted and sang the odd nursery rhyme. Not something anyone else wants to hear.

I sat him back in the pushchair on the way home as we said bye bye to the ducks and he turned and said 'I love you Nanny, thank you'. My heart melted and I could have cried on the spot as I suddenly realised that despite having spent a fair bit of time with him, this was probably the first time I had been truly present, not thinking about anything other than him and our time together.

The following morning, I looked in the mirror, really looked, whilst contemplating what had happened the day before. Did I even recognise myself? How had I let this happen? I had lost myself, lost one of my most precious values, family. I had been doing a sprint whilst running a marathon. No wonder I was struggling.

Back to the books, the course, the personal development I had been consuming. *If you don't make time for health then you will have to make time for illness* – I understand now.

Cardiac problems, not being present, I needed to change my practice and soon. I restarted some meditation, just a short, guided practice I had been recommended by Deepak Chopra. I found his voice very soothing, and it worked, his voice and words would allow me to breathe deeply and slowly, really taking in the air which seemed to open my heart and finally feel a pure sense of relaxation.

A sense of calm surrounded me for moments whilst in meditation. Calm that I never experience outside of this practice.

I invite you to ask yourself:

What do you do to experience TRUE relaxation?

Have you EVER experienced true relaxation?

What could change if you knew how to REALLY relax whenever you chose to?

Meditation evolved into more than just a relaxation technique for me—it has become a transformative experience, benefiting both my body and my mind. Beyond the physical sensations of calmness, I began to notice a shift in my mental state. Meditation has opened up space within my mind, allowing new thoughts, ideas and inspirations to flow in effortlessly.

As I continued my daily practice of setting aside 20 minutes for meditation, I found myself embracing it as a vital part of my routine. It wasn't always easy; I had to consciously prioritise this time and train myself to commit to it consistently. However, before long, meditation had become a non-negotiable aspect of my day.

The benefits are undeniable; when I skip a session, I can sense a subtle imbalance, a feeling of something missing from my inner equilibrium. I start to get irritable and listen more and more to that monkey chatter that increases as my anxious mind starts to sprint again.

People often think of meditation as slightly airy-fairy, yet many successful people in this world meditate.

Oprah Winfrey: The media mogul and philanthropist has been a longtime advocate for mindfulness and meditation. She has spoken openly about how meditation has helped her manage stress and stay grounded in her busy life.

Hugh Jackman: The actor, known for his roles in movies such as "X-Men" and "The Greatest Showman," has spoken about how meditation helps him stay centred and focused amidst the demands of his career.

Emma Watson: The British actress, best known for her role as Hermione Granger in the Harry Potter film series, has spoken about her interest in meditation and mindfulness. She has shared how these practices help her manage stress and stay grounded.

Richard Branson: The entrepreneur and founder of the Virgin Group has credited meditation with helping him stay focused and creative in his business ventures. He often advocates for the benefits of mindfulness and meditation in the workplace.

These individuals all highlight the widespread adoption of meditation practices across various fields and industries, demonstrating its benefits for enhancing well-being and performance. It's a practice that I think is misunderstood by many. When I first started, I believed I wasn't doing it correctly as I found it so difficult to sit still and 'clear my mind'. What I realised in time is that It's not about clearing your mind as such, it's about allowing the thoughts to flow through you like the wind through the trees.

Can anyone clear their mind completely? For me it's about taking control and not letting the monkey chatter take over. It's grounding, calming and contributes to overall inner strength.

Imagine your mind as a pond. Throughout the day, various thoughts, emotions and external stimuli create ripples on the surface of the pond, making it turbulent and cloudy. This turbulence represents stress, anxiety, and the chaos of daily life. Meditation is like settling the pond. When you sit in stillness, it's as if you allow the sediment to settle at the bottom, and the water becomes clearer. The ripples fade away, leaving a calm and serene surface. In this state, you can see to the depths of the pond, representing increased self-awareness, clarity of thought, and a peaceful mind.

Just as practising meditation regularly helps maintain the clarity of the pond, integrating meditation into my routine led to a calmer, more centred mind in the midst of life's storms.

Daily practices or habits can have a huge impact on your life and health. Old habits can be hard to break but with a mindset shift and consistency we can change the undesirable ones to habits that support who we would like to be and become.

Life consistently presents challenges, but consider the analogy of the gym. Several months ago, I began attending gym classes regularly. Initially, these sessions left me feeling incredibly sore the following day. However, after just a couple of weeks, I noticed a significant decrease in those day-two aches and pains. This transformation occurred because I remained consistent in my practice, allowing the muscles that initially experienced strain to heal and grow stronger. Similarly, my mental fitness underwent a parallel process. Just as physical stress and repair contribute to physical strength, the challenges we face in life stimulate mental growth and resilience.

True relaxation isn't just about rest—it's about presence. In the stillness of a walk with my grandson, I finally understood what it meant to be fully here, in the moment, without distraction. That moment became a catalyst for change. If I could lose myself in busyness and stress, I could also reclaim myself through awareness and intentionality. Meditation became my bridge back to balance, a daily practice that quietened the noise and reconnected me to what truly mattered. But as I began to reclaim my sense of purpose, I realised that change wasn't just something to embrace—it was something I needed to create. In the next chapter, I step beyond reflection and into action, leaving behind what no longer served me and stepping into a new path where impact, fulfilment, and transformation take centre stage.

CHAPTER 12

Echoes of Change

I have now left my role as a Matron. When I looked in that mirror, I no longer recognised the person I was. I had become disconnected; I was going through the motions and had started to feel dragged down by the negativity and conflict which I felt surrounded me. 'I've reached my limit,' I thought to myself, 'it's time for a change.' There was a dawning realisation that I was not where I was supposed to be, there was no fulfilment anymore, and without action nothing would change; in that moment the veil lifted.

With crystal-clear clarity, I now understood that I possessed the power to make a meaningful impact in a different realm. This clarity came partly due to an event I reflected on during the pandemic. I went into work at around 5:30 one morning to find three of our deployed nurses sitting silently in the coffee room looking very sad. I asked them about their night, and they proceeded to tell me how awful it had been. They had had four deaths and had felt useless. They told me how they had not been able to do anything and said the intensive care nurses had been literally running around. They had started to cry; I could see the pain inside them. I asked them a few questions: 'Did you wash the patients, did you brush their teeth and brush their hair, did you hold their hand?' They replied yes to all these things.

I went on to say to them that if they did nothing else other than those things whilst they were with us then I would be very happy and grateful for them being there, because the trained ITU nurses did not have time. If they had not been there the patients would have been alone.

I could see their expressions changing as I went on to explain that if one of their patients had been either of my parents, then I would have been very grateful for their input of care. It's not all about the drugs and equipment; the human everyday care they had given to these patients at a time their families were not able to is just as important. Just as I had discovered while feeding the ducks with my grandson, presence is the greatest gift we can give to another.

They looked at me a little confused and said they hadn't thought of it like that. I sincerely hope they went home and slept well that day, safe in the knowledge that they had done the best they could, which was enough.

Thinking about moments like this made me realise that I enjoy helping people overcome their fears, anxiety and daily stress. I believe I was put on this planet to support others. I have cared for my family, for patients, then staff, and now it is time to share my knowledge and experience to help others live a fulfilling life and realise their potential.

I hold a deep belief that there's purpose in every experience; it's simply a matter of gently questioning what life seeks to impart. Perspective, I've found, holds immense power in this journey. I see our world as a welcoming place, and I believe that as more individuals awaken to their true selves and the endless possibilities, our collective experience becomes richer.

I've come to understand that a truly fulfilling life revolves around three primary pillars: health, wealth, and relationships. While this notion isn't ground-breaking, it's essential to contemplate these aspects of existence. Take a moment to consider how you engage with each area, why you do so, and whether adjustments can enrich your experience.

Imagine your life as a delicate ecosystem, where health, wealth and relationships are the key components. Just as in nature, each element relies on the others to thrive, and when one is out of balance, it affects the entire system.

Health: Your physical and mental well-being form

the foundation of this ecosystem. When you prioritise your health, you have the energy, vitality and clarity of mind to pursue your goals and nurture your relationships. Without good health, your ability to enjoy life and achieve success in other areas is compromised.

Looking at health from a holistic position is imperative to overall mental, emotional and physical wellbeing.

There is a glaring irony when I consider health and the NHS, which is that due to the excessive hours and intense working environments, there are many health professionals out there sacrificing their own physical and mental health in order to do their job.

If you do not make time for health, you will have to make time for illness.

Wealth: This encompasses not only financial prosperity but also personal fulfilment and professional success. When you're financially stable and fulfilled in your career or endeavours, you have the resources to take care of your health and invest in meaningful relationships. However, an obsessive pursuit of wealth at the expense of health or relationships can lead to stress, burnout, and dissatisfaction.

Wealth can be considered in many ways. It can be seen as monetary, having a certain amount of cash in the bank or an income of a certain value or it can be considered as an abundance of something, anything. You can be wealthy in many ways. You can have a wealth of experience, love, relationships, food, or even just time.

Many people believe that to be wealthy they need a certain amount of money available to them. During the pandemic we had staff working ninety-plus hours a week consistently. Most nurses do extra shifts to top up their salary to live, but also to help their colleagues because, as we are all aware, there are not enough staff to cover the normal day to day running of a unit, never mind during these turbulent times.

They were paid for the extra shifts but, given the choice, I believe most of them would have worked as much despite the financial gain. Finances were not at the forefront of their minds.

Thus, I cannot imagine any of them would say that they became financially wealthy during this time. However, I do believe that the sense of meaning and purpose many of them experienced during this time, will have increased their sense of self-worth, aka inner wealth.

Wealth is most definitely an abundance of something. *Do we appreciate this, or is it just when something goes wrong that we realise with the benefit of hindsight what we had?* Joining the dots backwards is a fairly common phrase and if we do this, we often see what we had in terms of its value to us.

If you do not make time for abundance, you will have to make time for scarcity.

Relationships: Human connections are essential for

happiness and fulfilment. Healthy relationships provide support, love, and a sense of belonging. When your relationships are strong and nourishing, they contribute to your overall well-being and success. Conversely, neglecting or experiencing turmoil in your relationships can have a detrimental impact on your health and wealth.

One beautiful thing about working as a team through tough times and in intense circumstances is that strong relationships are forged quickly. I know that for many of my colleagues, the strength of these working relationships was the foundation which allowed them to get through the madness.

I have many different types of relationships in my life and they all seem to be determined by who I am at the time. Have you ever looked at your relationships from the perspective of your higher self and considered why they are so different?

If you do not make time for connection, you will have to make time for isolation.

Just like a well-balanced ecosystem, harmony between health, wealth and relationships is crucial for your overall happiness and fulfilment. When these areas are in sync, you experience a sense of wholeness and abundance in your life. If one area is neglected or in turmoil, it can throw off the balance and lead to feelings of stress, unhappiness, and discontent. Therefore, I strive to cultivate balance and harmony among these three pillars of life. By nurturing my health, fostering prosperity, and cultivating meaningful connections, I can create a solid foundation for a fulfilling and rewarding life journey.

We are all programmed from an early age to act and respond in a certain way. It is our internal programming that is running on autopilot that sometimes prevents us from seeing who we are showing up as. If we take the time to consider this and understand how our reality really works, then we can see quite clearly what we need to address in order to be who we would like to be.

I have shared one example of how my autopilot affected my health. I had not been prioritising my body and mind to support good health. Disease, or dis-ease, is often experienced because of imbalance.

Where are your scales tipping?

Change is rarely easy, but when the calling for transformation becomes louder than the fear of the unknown, we have no choice but to listen. Walking away from my role as a Matron wasn't just about leaving a job—it was about reclaiming my sense of purpose, rediscovering my voice, and choosing to live in alignment with what truly mattered. Through every experience, I had been preparing for this moment, learning that presence, care, and perspective hold more power than position or title. But stepping into a new path doesn't mean leaving behind who we are—it means embracing all the parts of our-

selves, the seen and unseen. In the next chapter, I reflect on the fluid nature of identity, exploring how we shift and adapt in different roles, and what it truly means to show up as our most authentic selves, no matter where life takes us.

CHAPTER 13

Bridges to Tomorrow

In the realm of personal development, I've come to recognise a profound truth: our identity is not fixed, but rather fluid, shaped by our surroundings and interactions. Much as a chameleon adapts its colour to blend seamlessly into its environment, we adjust our persona to fit the context we find ourselves in.

Consider this analogy: just as a skilled actor effortlessly embodies various characters on stage, we too possess the innate ability to adopt different roles in different situations. This adaptability is not a weakness, but rather a testament to our versatility and capacity for growth.

However, amidst this adaptability lies a profound question: What if we were to embrace our true selves unapologetically, regardless of our surroundings?

Would this be perceived as egotistical, or would it signify a newfound sense of authenticity?

In pondering this question, it's crucial to recognise that authenticity does not equate to rigidity. Rather, it embodies a deep sense of self-awareness and integrity, allowing us to navigate diverse environments while remaining true to our core values and beliefs.

During the pandemic I had many situations where I had to show up as my authentic self. I like to think I have integrity, but that was challenged many times as people thrust their demands on me in an unapologetic emotional chorus, which I knew was coming from a place of fear and their own need to please others around them.

If I did not stand up and explain how an intensive care unit runs, how the needs of the patients differed from other inpatients, and how the equipment and monitoring demanded expertise, then we would potentially have accepted many more patients than we could have coped with and everything would have become unsafe.

I remained steadfast in my response to the powers above me despite the pressure, as I knew I had to protect patients and the staff as much as possible.

I know for a fact though that my integrity was questioned by those below me. I often had conversations with staff who questioned many of the decisions I had made. However, I know any decisions I made came from a place of benevolence and that one thing, whether the decision turned out right or wrong, is what kept me on track and in doing the best I could.

A particular day comes to mind here. When life had settled post pandemic, we had a team leaders' meeting. During that meeting everyone was asked to share their thoughts. As the conversation went around the room one of the nurses pointed directly at me and spoke with anger and passion as she accused me of not being a part of the team. A tirade flowed from her as she just pointed and released all of her frustrations.

I sat still and listened until she was finished. Unsure of what to say or do, I merely thanked her for sharing her thoughts and suggested it was time for a break. The fifteen-minute break allowed me time to go to my office and take some very deep breaths. I wanted to cry and retaliate by defending my actions, but what purpose would that have served? I knew that everything I did was for them and the patients and there was no need to bring them into the world I had been living in. That would not have helped anyone and it was, in my opinion, my job to protect them from as much of the logistical, strategic pressure being put on us at the time, as possible. Should I defend myself or should I just let this go? I decided to let it go and accept that this was her opinion and not one that I was going to be able to change by expressing the challenges I had faced.

All I could do with this was offer the space for her to offload and listen. Hopefully some reflection followed. The day ended well but there is no doubt in my mind that many people felt this frustration for a number of reasons throughout this period.

Embodying our true selves may initially appear daunting, challenging the status quo of societal norms and expectations. Yet, it also offers a pathway to genuine connection and fulfilment, as we forge deeper, more authentic relationships based on mutual respect and understanding.

Ultimately, the journey towards authenticity is not a solitary endeavour but a collective exploration of self-discovery and growth. By embracing our true selves and showing up authentically, we not only honour our individuality but also inspire others to do the same, fostering a more genuine and empathetic world.

A classic example of this is when I was 'the daughter' at the nursing home. I became submissive at times, believing others around me knew what they were doing better than I did. I allowed myself to feel 'less than' which is a limiting belief I have struggled with over many years.

Why do we do this, why do we limit ourselves? No one person is above or below you. Everyone has value and everyone matters.

I questioned my knowledge and suppressed my opinion until I exploded into a thousand pieces and collapsed, sobbing over my dad. If I had been more confident to be me, to communicate and build an understanding relationship with those around me in the home, this might not have happened. I did myself an injustice that ultimately affected my own dad.

At work, I was decisive, a warrior to my tribe. I was strong and determined to fight for every tiny detail that would help them carry out their work in the best way possible. Yet, did my team see this, did they know how I was fighting for them with those above me? Did the people above me appreciate where I was coming from and why I was doing what I was?

At home, I was Jekyll & Hyde. My family would tell you I am strong and look to me for answers, but they also saw me as either a volcano, boiling inside and ready to erupt at any time or an overly sensitive being who cried at the drop of a hat.

In each of these settings (during the pandemic, at work, with the family) I was presenting differently. Why? Because, as I said earlier, we are designed to adapt to the environment around us. So the difference in the way I was showing up is divine, an incredible aspect of being human.

If I look at each of those situations, however different I may seem to be, there is something which remains the same in each. Regardless of what situation I find myself in, there is always a sense of my true self, that part of me which has been the same since I was a child, the eternal part of me.

The challenge people have is that they rarely identify

with that eternal part of themselves, and instead allow the world around them to shape their identity. This creates attachment to something temporary, and when the ever-changing outer world moves things around, they feel a sense of loss as an aspect of their identity changes or ceases to exist. The common response to this is anger and resistance as a defence mechanism against a feeling of 'losing themselves'.

The first step toward a more authentic identity is inner inquiry into the relationship you have with yourself, as it is the first one you need to recognise and the most important one to nurture.

You can't give from an empty cup. Looking back, my relationship with myself was turbulent and not one that had much self-love.

If you don't have a good relationship with yourself, then how can you have a good one with others?

> *Our identities shift and adapt, moulded by the environments we navigate—but beneath it all, there is a core self, unchanging and true. The challenge is not in choosing one version over another, but in aligning each role with authenticity and integrity. It takes courage to stand firm in who we are while adapting to the ever-changing world around us. Yet when we embrace this fluidity without losing sight of our values, we find a deeper sense of purpose and inner peace. In the next*

chapter, we delve into the power of possibility, exploring how understanding our inner archetypes—Warrior, Magician, Lover, and Sovereign—can guide us through the turbulent waters of life, helping us steer our course with clarity, resilience, and purpose.

CHAPTER 14

The Power of Possibility

Back to my river of life:

Imagine navigating the waters of life in a small boat. This boat represents the relationship with yourself. In a turbulent relationship the waves are unpredictable and stormy. The boat is tossed about and it feels like you are constantly battling the elements. The waves represent self-doubt, inner conflict and negative talk. Each wave shakes the boat, making it challenging to find stability. The more the storm rages, the harder it is to stay on course.

In this analogy, finding inner peace and a healthy relationship with oneself is akin to learning to navigate stormy waters. It involves developing skills to steady the boat, understanding the patterns of the waves (thoughts and emotions), and gradually learning to navigate through the challenges with resilience.

Just as a skilled sailor can navigate through rough seas with grace, cultivating self-awareness, self-compassion and positive self-talk can help you navigate the storms within, leading to a more stable and harmonious relationship with yourself.

An understanding of different personalities or relationship archetypes can help us navigate all our relationships. Archetypes are a person's blueprint, their go-to personality, of which there are four main types: Warrior, Magician, Lover, Sovereign. We are all capable of showing up as more than one archetype. If you think back to the events in this book I have shown up to some degree as each of the four archetypes at one time or another.

The Warrior

The Warrior represents a figure characterised by strength, courage, and a commitment to protect and uphold values or ideals. This archetype is often associated with resilience, discipline and a sense of duty. The warrior faces challenges and adversities with bravery, demonstrating both physical and moral fortitude. They are driven by a purpose, whether it be defending others, fighting for justice, or overcoming personal obstacles. The warrior embodies the principles of honour and sacrifice, striving to achieve their goals through determination and perseverance.

My experience:

The Warrior archetype emerged in me during the moments when standing firm was the only way to protect those who depended on me. Whether it was my staff or my patients, I felt a deep sense of duty to safeguard their well-being, even when it meant challenging authority or risking being misunderstood. My strength as a Warrior was rooted not just in my willingness to confront adversity but in my unwavering commitment to do what was right.

I recall instances where decisions from higher management felt disconnected from the realities on the ground. These were moments that demanded courage—to push back, to question, and to advocate for what I believed to be in the best interests of my team and patients. While this might have been seen as argumentative or obstructive by some, my intention was clear: to protect and uphold the values of care, compassion, and fairness that defined our work.

As a Warrior, I found myself standing at the frontline of more than just the pandemic—I was defending the emotional and physical well-being of those around me. My resilience and moral fortitude allowed me to navigate these challenges with determination, even when the path was unclear. The Warrior archetype isn't about seeking conflict but about facing it head-on when necessary, driven by a purpose greater than oneself.

This sense of honour guided me through difficult conversations and hard-fought battles. It reminded me that true strength lies not in avoiding challenges but in confronting them with integrity and conviction. Through these moments, I upheld my duty to my team, my patients, and my own principles, embodying the spirit of a Warrior who fights not for glory, but for what is just and right.

The Magician:

The Magician symbolises transformation, wisdom, and the power to effect change through insight and innovation. This figure is often associated with mystical knowledge and the ability to unlock hidden potentials within oneself and others. The magician harnesses the forces of the universe, using imagination and intuition to manifest new realities and guide others through periods of transition. They are seen as visionaries and catalysts for change, bridging the gap between the known and the unknown, and bringing about profound shifts through their understanding of deeper truths and hidden possibilities.

My experience:

My role as a Magician became evident in moments that

demanded transformation, creativity and unwavering vision. One of the most striking examples was creating the antechambers for our unit during the pandemic. With limited resources and no clear precedent to follow, we harnessed our imagination to envision what could be. We transformed ideas into reality, crafting solutions that not only addressed immediate challenges but also set a foundation for safer practices in unprecedented circumstances. This was innovation born out of necessity, driven by a belief in possibilities yet unseen.

On a personal level, I acted as my own Magician, transforming grief and hardship into a wellspring of resilience and wisdom. Through practices like journaling and self-reflection, I uncovered the hidden potential within myself, turning pain into a catalyst for profound growth. This transformation not only carried me through the most difficult moments but also inspired me to step into the role of mentor and trainer, guiding others through their own periods of transition and change.

In every instance, the Magician archetype guided me to see beyond what was, to imagine what could be, and to manifest a reality shaped by wisdom, vision, and an unwavering belief in the power of transformation.

The Lover

The Lover archetype embodies passion, connection and

the pursuit of deep, meaningful relationships. This figure is characterised by their capacity for empathy, intimacy and the appreciation of beauty and harmony in life. The Lover is driven by a profound desire to connect with others on an emotional and sensory level, seeking to nurture and sustain relationships through love, compassion, and creativity. They thrive on creating and experiencing joy, and their presence often inspires a sense of unity and fulfilment in both themselves and those around them. The lover archetype emphasises the importance of vulnerability, emotional expression, and the transformative power of love.

My experience:

The Lover archetype came alive in the moments when connection, empathy and compassion were needed most. As a leader during the pandemic, I saw first-hand the emotional toll that the crisis was taking on my team. Every conversation, every moment of listening, became an opportunity to embody the Lover's essence. I opened myself to their vulnerability, offering a safe space for them to express their fears, frustrations, and grief.

I remember sitting with a staff member who was overwhelmed by the weight of their responsibilities, their voice shaking as they described the pressure of being on the front line. In that moment, I wasn't just a matron; I was a listener, a confidante, and a source of solace. My drive to relieve their internal suffering came not from a sense of duty alone but from a deep well of compassion—a Lover's desire to nurture and sustain the emotional well-being of those around me.

This capacity for empathy and vulnerability didn't only serve my team—it transformed me. Each act of love, compassion, and support strengthened my own resolve, reminding me of the transformative power of connection. It was in these moments that I realised love is not only an emotion but a force for healing, uniting, and inspiring us all to move forward together.

The Sovereign

The Sovereign archetype represents leadership, authority and the embodiment of stability and order. This figure is characterised by the ability to guide and rule with wisdom, responsibility and a sense of justice. The sovereign provides direction, ensures the well-being of their domain, and upholds principles of fairness and integrity. They are seen as stabilisers and decision-makers, balancing the needs of their people or realm with a strategic vision. The sovereign archetype embodies qualities of confidence, stewardship, and the capacity to inspire respect and loyalty through their principled leadership and unwavering commitment to their role.

My experience:

The Sovereign archetype became my guiding force during the most critical moments of the pandemic. As a leader, I was responsible not only for navigating the chaos but for maintaining stability and ensuring the well-being of everyone under my care. Each decision I made required a delicate balance—responding to the demands of strategic management while prioritising the needs of my team and patients. The Sovereign in me understood that leadership meant not just authority but stewardship, ensuring that no one was overlooked, regardless of their position or role.

I recall meticulously planning every aspect of the unit's response, from logistics to morale. It wasn't enough to follow directives from above—I had to translate those strategies into actions that made sense for the reality on the ground. That meant considering the physical, emotional and professional needs of my team and making decisions that would sustain us all through the toughest days.

In those moments, I saw myself not just as a leader but as a protector of my team's well-being. I tried to ensure that every individual, whether they were a nurse, doctor, or cleaner, felt valued and supported. The Sovereign archetype compelled me to lead with fairness and integrity. I knew that unity and stability would be our greatest strengths in the face of uncertainty.

Through it all, I strived to embody the qualities of a true Sovereign: calm amidst chaos, decisiveness in uncertainty, and compassion in authority. These principles not only guided me in supporting my team but also helped me maintain a vision of hope and resilience, inspiring loyalty and respect when it mattered most.

Having an understanding of people's archetypes can really help you to become conscious of where they are coming from and also how to communicate with them in a way they will hear you.

While we each have all four archetypal personality blueprints within us, there will be one which we resonate with the most; our default setting if you will.

For many, the qualities of the other three archetypes can seem unclear or even contradictory, often resulting in misunderstanding and tension in our interactions. Without taking the time to explore and understand these archetypes, we risk misalignment with the majority of people we encounter—possibly up to 75% of them.

Why does this happen?

Each of us is shaped by our own unique archetypal blueprint that influences how we behave and how we communicate and respond to the world around us. These traits, preferences and patterns can differ significantly between archetypes, making it easy to misinterpret others or struggle to understand our own emotions and actions.

Gaining clarity about your own archetype is essential to making sense of why you feel and act the way you do in different situations. It allows you to recognise the archetypal influences guiding your thoughts and emotions in the moment. With this understanding, you can approach both your inner world and your relationships with greater awareness, empathy, and intention.

This follows a simple formula that explains what happens when there is a misunderstanding of the archetype:

Confusion > Conflict > Breakdown > Suffering

Think back to that colleague who you just couldn't understand, or that intimate partner who seemed great at first before apparently turning into a monster. The examples are endless, so let me just say this: 90%+ of all breakdowns and suffering you've ever experienced in relationships stem from archetypal confusion.

This simple formula underscores the importance of understanding all four archetypes. Without investing the time to reduce archetypal confusion, we inevitably end up investing time in navigating archetypal suffering. This principle applies not only to how we engage with others in the external world but also to how we interact with ourselves internally.

In my own experience, I've seen how archetypal confusion can create significant internal struggles. While the warrior archetype isn't my natural default, I found myself fully embodying it during a particularly challenging time—a necessity given the situation. What followed was an internal breakdown that vividly illustrates how archetypal suffering can manifest within us when we are pushed into roles that don't align with our inherent nature. Let me take you through this moment to shed light on how these dynamics can play out.

There came a point during the relentless chaos of the pandemic when the strength I prided myself on as a Warrior began to falter. I had been fighting so hard, pushing back against decisions I felt were unjust, advocating for my staff's well-being, and shielding my patients from the ripple effects of strained resources. Every battle felt like it mattered, and yet, the weight of it all began to feel unbearable.

One particular night, after another heated exchange with management over staffing shortages, I found myself alone in the break room, staring blankly at the wall. The adrenaline that had driven me through so many battles was gone, replaced by a hollow sense of defeat. My body felt heavy, my mind clouded. I realised I had nothing left to give, not because the fight was over, but because I was drained from fighting so hard for so long.

In that moment, the Warrior in me cracked. I questioned whether my efforts were making any difference, whether I was truly protecting those I cared about or simply exhausting myself in a futile struggle. The exhaustion wasn't just physical—it was emotional, mental, and spiritual. I felt the creeping doubt of whether I could keep going, whether I had the strength to continue being the shield and the sword for my team and my patients.

But even in that breakdown, there was a lesson. As I sat there, tears I didn't know I had been holding back began to fall, releasing the pressure that had been building for months. It was a reminder that even Warriors need rest, that strength isn't about never breaking—it's about finding the courage to acknowledge when you've reached your limits. It was in this moment of vulnerability that I began to understand the balance between fighting for others and caring for myself, a lesson that would ultimately shape the way I approached my role moving forward.

1. Confusion
This is the initial stage where the archetype begins to falter. For the Warrior, confusion might arise when they question the effectiveness of their actions or feel uncertain about the impact of their efforts. In the example above, confusion is reflected in the doubt about whether the constant battles are making any difference.

2. Conflict

As confusion grows, it leads to an internal or external conflict. For the Warrior, this could be an internal struggle between their sense of duty and their physical or emotional limits, or an external battle with the systems or people they're pushing against. The example captures this through the heated exchanges with management and the internal questioning of whether the fight is worth continuing.

3. Breakdown

The conflict becomes overwhelming, leading to a point of collapse. This is the moment when the archetype's strength is temporarily lost, and they are forced to confront their vulnerability. Again, in the example the scene in the break room where exhaustion overtakes me, and the tears signal a release of the bottled-up pressure.

4. Suffering

In the aftermath of the breakdown, there's a period of suffering—emotional, mental, or physical. However, this stage also offers the possibility of transformation and growth. In this example suffering teaches the lesson that even I am not invincible, and self-care is a critical part of resilience.

We are fluid, ever-changing beings, adapting to our environments and roles—sometimes seamlessly, sometimes painfully. Whether as a Warrior, Magician, Lover, or Sovereign, each archetype represents a piece of who we are, shaping how we show up in the world. But when we become too attached to a single identity, we risk losing sight of the balance between them all. The path to true self-awareness isn't about clinging to one role—it's about learning when to step into each, and when to let go.

In the next chapter, I explore how this awareness can unlock new possibilities, transforming the way we navigate life's challenges and opportunities. Because when we understand ourselves, we don't just survive the storms—we learn to sail through them.

CHAPTER 15

Embracing the Journey

As I sit here reflecting on the path that has unfolded before me, I am struck by the profound realisation that every twist, every heartbreak and every moment of doubt was part of a larger tapestry woven with threads of resilience, growth, and transformation. The journey was never about reaching a single destination but about uncovering the layers within myself, layer by layer, breath by breath.

Grief taught me the fragility of life, but it also revealed an unexpected strength. The loss of my father, the relentless demands of the pandemic and the heartache etched into those long days and nights became mirrors reflecting not just pain but the depth of love, connection, and the unyielding spirit within me. I learned that healing isn't a linear process. It comes in waves—sometimes gentle, sometimes fierce—but always with lessons hidden beneath the surface.

The tools I once saw as lifelines—journaling, reflection, personal development practices—evolved into more than just coping mechanisms. They became the pillars upon which I rebuilt my life. Each journal entry was not just ink on paper; it was a declaration of survival, a testament to the power of vulnerability, and an acknowledgment that even in the darkest times, there is light to be found within.

This journey has shown me that resilience isn't about bouncing back to who we were before our struggles. It's about integrating our experiences, honouring our growth, and embracing the new versions of ourselves that emerge from the ashes of our old identities. The person writing these words is not the same person who began this journey—and that's the greatest gift of all.

As I close this chapter, I carry forward not just the memories of loss and hardship, but the wisdom born from those experiences. Life will continue to unfold with its inevitable challenges, but now I meet it with an open heart, grounded in the knowledge that I am capable of navigating whatever comes my way.

In the pages that follow, the epilogue serves as both a reflection and an invitation—a reminder that while one story may end, another always begins. And as we step into the unknown, may we do so with courage, compassion, and an unwavering belief in our ability to rise, again and again.

EPILOGUE:

The Journey Continues

In the wake of unimaginable challenges, we often find ourselves standing at the precipice of profound change, our spirits tested and our hearts heavy. As I reflect on my journey through the trials of the COVID-19 pandemic, I see not just the darkness of loss and adversity but also the transformative light that emerged from it. This book is not merely a recounting of my experiences but a testament to the extraordinary strength of the human spirit.

The pandemic, with its relentless demands and personal heartaches, pushed me to the limits of my endurance, yet it also illuminated a path to profound personal growth. The pain of losing my dad, grappling with professional responsibilities, and confronting my own vulnerabilities were not the end of my story but the beginning of a new chapter. Through these trials, I discovered the power of resilience, the importance of self-compassion, and the transformative impact of inner work.

Since writing this book, my journey has continued to evolve. Recognising the need for rest and change, I stepped into a more strategic role within healthcare. This decision wasn't just about shifting gears; it was about acknowledging the importance of balance, growth, and renewal. This role has given me the space to learn, reflect, and contribute in a different way—shaping the future of healthcare not from the frontlines, but from a perspective that allows me to influence and advocate for systemic change.

Even now, the work of self-discovery continues. There are moments when I still struggle, but those struggles are no longer overwhelming. The dark places I once found myself in are now temporary spaces I visit, never places where I linger. The tools I've gained—reflection, meditation, and personal development—remain my compass, guiding me through each challenge with clarity and resolve.

This journey has been one of ongoing discoveries. I move forward with hope, courage and integrity, striving every day to align with my true self and inspire others to do the same. I believe deeply that when we live authentically and with purpose, we unlock not only our own potential but also the ability to uplift those around us.

My message is this: Transformation is a journey, not a destination. If you find yourself feeling lost, unfulfilled or overwhelmed, know that you have within you the power to change your course. The same principles that carried me through the storm—resilience, self-reflection and the courage to embrace change—are available to you. Every step forward, no matter how small, brings you closer to a life that resonates with your deepest desires.

The world is still healing, and so are we. In this time of recovery, there lies an extraordinary opportunity for renewal—not just for ourselves, but for the communities and systems we are part of. Together, we can transcend the limitations of our past and build a future filled with purpose, passion, and fulfilment.

If you're ready to embark on your own journey of transformation, I am here to walk alongside you. As a mentor, guide and fellow traveller on this path, I offer my experiences and insights to help you navigate your way. The lessons of this book are not just mine—they are universal truths that remind us of the resilience within us all.

Let us honour that resilience, not as a response to adversity alone, but as the proactive power for positive change. Embrace your journey of self-discovery, let it illuminate your path, and know that you are never alone in this process. Reach out, take that first step, and together we can forge a future where we not only survive, but thrive.

Here's to the power of resilience, the promise of

transformation, and the unwavering commitment to living a life of authenticity and purpose. May we all find our way to a brighter, more fulfilling tomorrow—and may we carry with us the courage to help others do the same.